MW00615012

YOGA, SEX AND HAPPINESS

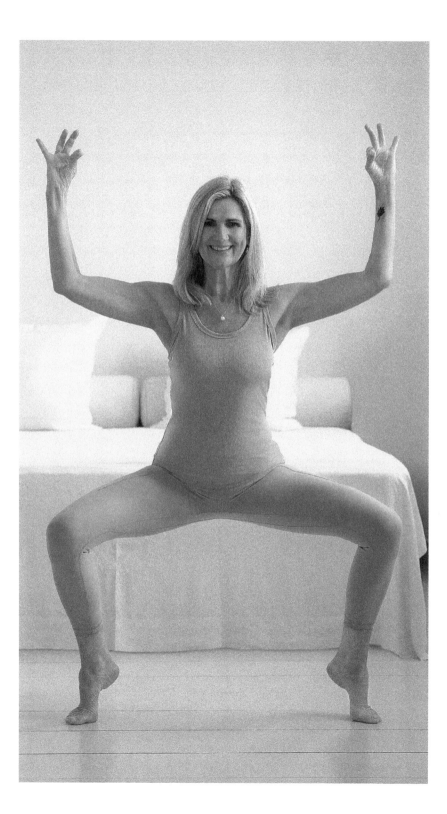

CAROLIN-MARIE ROTH

YOGA, SEX AND HAPPINESS

The smart guide to better health

PHOTOGRAPHY BY EVA LINDNER
ILLUSTRATIONS BY JOEY GURDON

FOR MY LOVELY YOGA STUDENTS,
PAST AND PRESENT.

CONTENTS

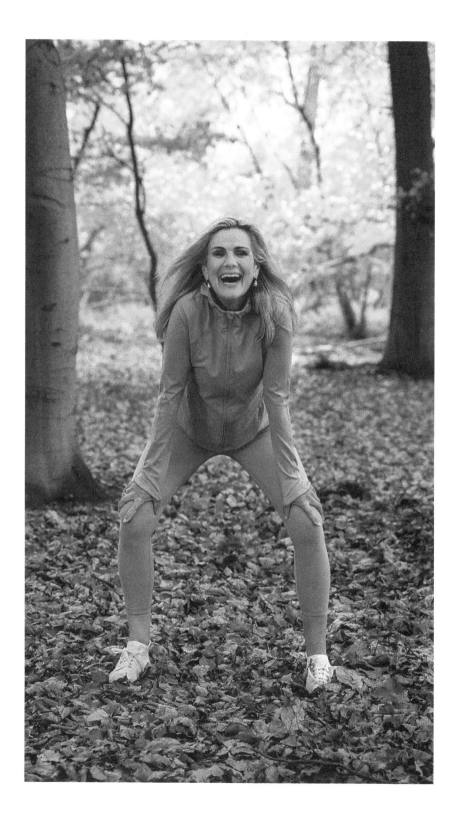

The beginning

*"Love you will find only where
you may show yourself weak
without provoking strength."* [1]

Theodor W. Adorno (Philosopher)

W hen people first meet me, they see a tall, slender blonde and automatically assume that I am the epitome of 'good health', but little do they know that my early childhood years in post-war Germany consisted of chaos, neglect and emotional abuse. Unloved and abandoned is not an easy situation for any child and, as a teenager, it was yoga that helped me to survive. It continues to support me to this day. After 50 years of practice, I am still learning that I cannot change things happening around me, but I can control how I react towards them.

I always wanted to write this book about yoga, hoping to provide a toolbox of sorts. Eventually, when the pandemic hit, leaving us all isolated during a time of uncertainty, I began my writing process – and it turned out to be quite a journey!

Throughout 23 chapters you will find detailed exercises that can assist you to deal with anger, anxiety, back pain, constipation, eating disorders, a fat belly, fibromyalgia, flatulence, getting old, hair loss, hangovers, happiness, insomnia, the menopause, osteoporosis, panic attacks, queefs, reflux, sex, stress, tennis elbow, tinnitus and weight loss.

The book is written in a modular format, so you can dip in and out of the chapters that are relevant to you. Each chapter has a range of yoga poses and some further tips. The postures are developed from my own practice, which is influenced by all different yoga schools, such as *Iyengar*, *Kundalini* and *Sivananda*.

The exercises are not particularly tough or demanding; they are simply what I know worked best to manage my health, first as a teenager, then as a grown woman and especially now that I am a grandmother. At the start of each exercise section, I suggest some optional props that can be used for ease and comfort, but all the exercises can be done equally effectively without props. For a list of props, see p.333.

I have poured my whole life into this book, in the hope that it can give you some ideas and support for your own journey. It should, at the very least, help you to ask the right questions when seeking advice from health professionals. The more informed you are, the easier it can be for your GP to help you.

My first ever interaction with yoga was around 1973, in the USA, where I lived with my uncle and his family. I watched 'Lilias Yoga and You', a television show hosted by Lilias Folan, North America's 'First Lady of Yoga'. Her simple yoga routines, which I practised religiously day and night, gave me structure, stability and comfort.

Then, I remember my early yoga sessions in Düsseldorf, Germany, during my university years. We had to meet in private houses as there were no yoga studios. My fellow yogis at the time were the musicians Ralf Hütter and Florian Schneider-Esleben, best known as the founding members of the electronic band Kraftwerk. Another yoga friend was one of the producers of Electric Music and Rheingold, Lothar

Manteuffel. There seemed to be a special connection between music, yoga and Germans searching for a better life.

Before I became a British Wheel of Yoga teacher 20 years ago, I used to work as a TV presenter and producer for RTL in Luxemburg and Germany. Throughout my TV career, I met and interviewed all kinds of famous and interesting people, but behind the glittery TV world I always craved for a family of my own and a life in London.

When my husband Jörg and I sold our London-based TV production company, we used some of our profits to found and run an award-winning charity, My Life Films, training young filmmakers to produce personalised films for people living with dementia. Today, we are still trustees of this charity and have since overseen the launch of the world's first streaming platform for people with cognitive needs, My Life TV – a kind of 'Netflix for Dementia' – all non-profit.

Besides our charity work, we co-own two Caribbean restaurants in East London called Rhythm Kitchen, which is 'one for the bucket list' according to the press. We like to keep busy and are lucky enough to live in leafy Richmond-upon-Thames, enjoying the beauty of our neighbourhood with our 3 grown-up daughters, 2 baby granddaughters and our labradoodle, Bowie.

So, a happy ending after all? Well, it's always work in progress. Nothing is guaranteed, but I try my best and go with the flow … and yoga helps with that too. I hope that *Yoga, Sex and Happiness* will help, inspire and encourage you on your own path and journey.

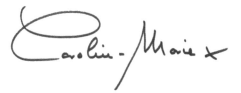

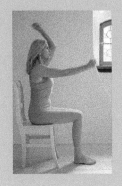

Anger

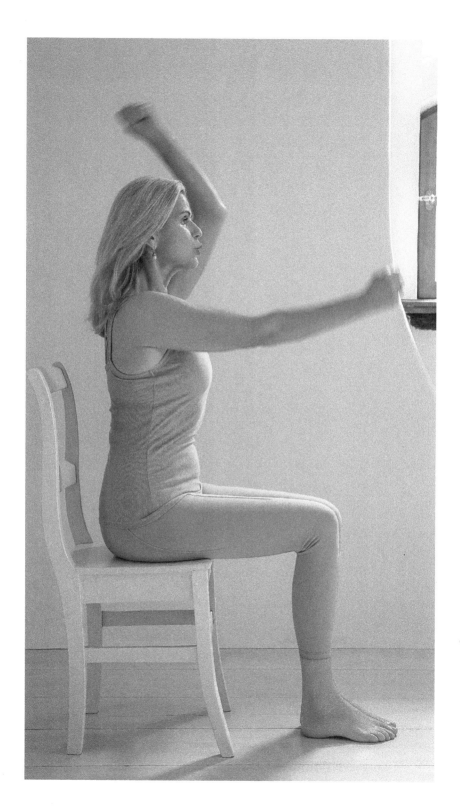

Anger

"You can survive with anger,
but you can't live with it forever." [1]

Ariel Dorfman (Human Rights Activist)

Everyone has the right to be angry … angry about politics, greed, inequality, injustice and cruelty. There are so many things in life that we are entitled to feel angry about.

As a child, I was angry with my alcoholic father and with myself for believing and hoping that one day he would overcome his addiction. Sadly, he never did, but the anger I felt at that time helped and motivated me to survive his abuse and eventually to thrive. That took willpower and a change of environment. I left Germany, my home, when I was 15 years old and moved in with relatives in the USA. Even though I felt lonely and homesick, I was determined to turn my life around and finish my school education.

Anger often is associated with destruction, but it also can be a force for good and change. Therefore, don't feel you must subdue your anger because you think it is not an appropriate or constructive emotion to have. Suppressing anger can lead to physical and mental stress and has long been suspected to have adverse health effects.[2] Research shows that people who are closed off from their emotions increase their chance of premature death, as well as the risk of having cancer.[3]

Yet, expressing anger can become a problem when it gets out of control and harms you or the people around you. Ideally, you will learn how to articulate *and* channel your anger at the same time.

There are yoga movements that allow you to do just that: to express *and* to manage your anger. Simple exercises that can help you to let off steam. Be prepared to make some noise, and clench and throw your fists – and all this without harming yourself or anyone else.

My favourite exercise to regulate my emotions is to turn into a roaring lion. *Simhagarjanasana* is a classic yoga posture that can unblock the *Vishuddha Chakra*, your throat and neck energy centre (see p.329). A free-flowing neck chakra can help to improve your communication, thus avoiding misunderstandings, anger and frustration.

During the Roaring Lion Pose, your eyes roll up to the point between your eyebrows, the seat of your *Ajna Chakra* (see p.330), the so-called 'third eye'. This chakra is the seat of intuition and wisdom but also the seat of anger. When your *Ajna Chakra* is working well, you feel alert and insightful, but when this chakra is blocked you can feel irritable and angry.

Another tool to manage your anger is the fire breath, which is an important element of *Kundalini Yoga*, a yoga school that is characterised by movement with the breath. The Breath of Fire is a rapid, rhythmic and energising breath, with a cleansing effect on your body and mind. This exercise can last up to 3 minutes, and you should clench your hands throughout. Making fists can stimulate your brain and help you to find your inner cool and calm. Clenching the right hand can activate the left, more analytical side of your brain, whereas clenching the left hand activates the more emotional, right side of your brain.[4]

Also, don't forget about good, old-fashioned forgiveness, which can be such a powerful tool. If you allow anger and negativity to crowd out positive feelings, you might find yourself overwhelmed by bitterness. But if you can forgive someone, you can both learn from the situation. The best yoga exercises to soften and to learn how to let go are forward bends, such as the seated one shown in this chapter.

For more anger-channelling exercises, look at the Reflux chapter (see p.253). People who experience heartburn are often prone to feel anger more than others and the recommended reflux exercises can help.

Anger often is associated with destruction, but it also can be a force for good and change.

EXERCISES

Roaring Lion Pose
(Simhagarjanasana)

Whenever you feel tension and anger rising, try this exercise. Given its expressive nature, you may prefer to practise it privately rather than in public!

This pose opens your throat chakra and cleanses your vocal cords, as well as releasing tension in your neck and shoulders. Your throat might feel sore afterwards, but overall you will feel great and a sense of relief.

● **Kneel on the floor** or sit on a chair with your knees apart. Place your hands on your knees. Take a few in- and out-breaths with your eyes closed.

● **Then, take a deep breath in,** hold your breath, open your eyes and splay your fingers like the sharpened claws of a wild cat, and roll your eyes up.

● **Now, breathe out loudly** through your mouth with a roaring 'Ha' sound and stick out your tongue as far as possible, while still breathing out.

● **Relax, close your eyes** and take a couple of normal in- and out-breaths again.

● **Repeat the loud and roaring lion breath** up to 5 times. You will instantly feel a release in your neck and throat area.

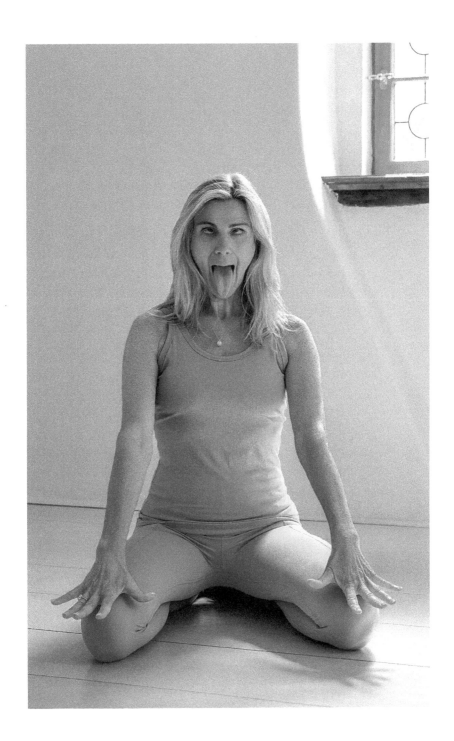

Fist of Anger and Breath of Fire

Yogis believe that hand gestures, *Mudras*, such as clenching your hands and squeezing your thumbs, can help to channel and shift energies from what you might be experiencing to how you want to feel. So, yoga can help you to bring the fire (*Agni*) back into balance with the other elements such as earth (*Prithvi*), water (*Jal*), air (*Vayu*) and space (*Akasha*).

The Fist of Anger and Breath of Fire is best practised when your stomach and bowels are empty, typically early in the morning. If you feel lightheaded during the exercise, reduce your practice to just 1 minute and do not hold your breath at the end.[5]

Caution: Do not practise this exercise if you are pregnant, or if you are suffering from high blood pressure, heart disease, any respiratory conditions or vertigo.

● **Sit comfortably on a chair** or on the floor, with your spine straight. Bring your thumbs inside your fists (*Matsya Mudra*), extending your arms up towards the ceiling. Now, think about something or someone that makes you feel angry. Keep squeezing your thumbs throughout the exercise.

● **Then, starting with your left arm,** do backstrokes with both your arms over the top of your head, while breathing in through your nose and out through pursed lips (your mouth is formed like an 'O'). (See photo, p.16.)

● **Breathe in quick and sharply** through your nose and breathe out forcefully through your mouth as you move your lifted arms forwards and backwards above your head. Your belly button is moving with each in- and out-breath. If you feel a bit dizzy, slow down; otherwise try to practise at the same speed for 3 minutes.

● **When finished, keep both of your arms up** and over your head, interlace your fingers and turn your palms upwards. Breathe in and hold your breath for a couple of seconds.

● **To end, release both your arms** and enjoy this rush of new and hopefully positive energy. Repeat the exercise once more.

MODIFICATION
At the end of your fire breath practice, keep your arms lifted, open your palms, spread your fingers apart and scream at the top of your lungs for a few seconds. Then, slowly release your arms down by your sides and take a few moments to sit quietly and observe how you feel. Has anything shifted? Do you feel lighter? Do you feel more empowered? Does your throat hurt? How did it feel to give yourself permission to scream?

Shift energies from
what you might be
experiencing to what
you want to feel.

Seated Forward Bend
(Paschimottanasana)

This yoga exercise is rather passive because you allow gravity to stretch you, releasing tension and inducing relaxation.[6] A forward bend can help you to cool down feelings of anger and is particularly enjoyable when practising with a yoga bolster or a large cushion.

● **Start by sitting on the floor** with your legs extended out in front of you.

● **If you can't sit up straight,** then sit on a block or a book.

● **Place a bolster or cushion onto your straight legs.** If you do not have a cushion or bolster, bend your legs slightly.

● **As you inhale, lengthen your spine** and lift both arms with your palms facing each other. As you exhale, fold forwards from your hips so that your upper body comes over your legs and your arms and your head can rest on the bolster. If you are not using a bolster, keeping your legs slightly bent, bend forwards – making sure you are bending from the hips. Breathe in and say 'Yes' to something you want to believe in, e.g., hope. As you breathe out, tell yourself to let go of something you want relief from, e.g., your anger.

● **Do not force anything.** Willpower won't help you in forward bends but letting go will. Think forward rather than down as you keep elongating your upper body.

● **If your head does not reach the bolster,** either increase the height of the cushion or turn the bolster lengthways and rest your head against the small side. Hold this position for as long as it is comfortable.

Willpower won't help you
in forward bends, but
letting go will.

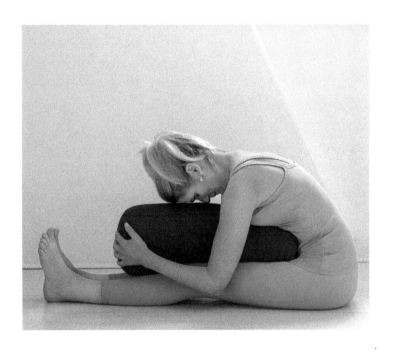

The Circle of Fire

Imagine that someone you feel close to annoys you and you find yourself in a heated confrontation, feeling furious and angry. Then, instead of fighting you unexpectedly stop arguing in mid-sentence and turn away from your partner without announcing it.

● **Physically turn your back to the person** you are arguing with, without any announcement; just turn around, don't say a word and close your eyes. Visualise a circle of fire, or you can call it a circle of anger, with you standing right in the middle of it.

● **Imagine that your feet start burning** and you can feel the heat crawling up your legs. But then concentrate on your breath. Focus on a deep and even in- and out-breath where you partially close the glottis in-between your vocal cords, developing a soft snoring sound. This deep, slow and even *Ujjayi Breath* (see p.84) can enact physical changes in your brain that can help you to shift your emotional state. Stay with the breath for at least a minute, zoning out from what is going on around you.

● **Eventually, leave the circle of fire** – just imagine literally stepping out of it.

● **Now that you are outside the circle** with your eyes open again, turn around and look at your partner. Notice, that there is less anger, no more raised voices and hopefully a more relaxed attitude on both sides.

● **If your partner bursts out laughing** when you turn around, just join in. Remember that nothing works faster to calm anger than a good laugh. Laughter (see p.171) can shift perspectives, allowing you to see any situation in a more realistic, less threatening light.[7]

FURTHER TIPS

● **Try less black-and-white thinking!** By avoiding this pattern, you can reduce anger. Overgeneralising often makes a situation seem worse than it really is.

● **Stop making assumptions.** We assume that people do not like us, lie to us, etc. The problem with making these assumptions is that we often believe they are true. So how to avoid making assumptions? Simply ask questions ● and make sure that the communication is clear. You will not always like what you hear, but at least you are not angry because you assumed something that is not true.

● **Stop taking everything personally.** Often people say hurtful things that cause anger. Remember that what others do or say is not necessarily because of you. Often it is a projection of their own reality, not yours.[8]

● **Try to replace anger** with assertiveness. Assertive people will try to get their needs met without hurting anyone else. Assertiveness is the middle ground between being pushy and being a pushover.

● **Start punching things** (not people) like a cushion or a punching ball with the face of the person who you really dislike and who angers you.

● **Scream,** ideally not at someone but when alone in a room with loud music on. Screaming can trigger feel-good hormones, endorphins, which can have a positive effect on your mental state.[9]

● **If nothing seems to make a difference** and you need urgent help and are in the UK, call 111 and ask for support. Or contact the charity Mind, www.mind.org.uk, for practical suggestions on how to cope with anger and where to go for help.

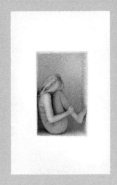

Anxiety

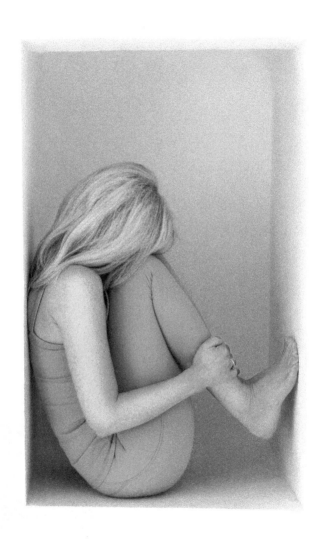

Anxiety

"If the promise of yoga on mental health was found in a drug, it would be the bestselling medication worldwide." [1]

Dr. P. Murali Doraiswamy (Scientist)

have been anxious for most of my life, but I never wanted anyone to see or feel my worries or my weakness. My biggest fear as a child was not being good enough, not worthy of being loved. I tried so hard to please my beautiful but narcissistic mum in the hope of getting some acknowledgement and warmth.

As a teenager, my main anxiety was fear of loss, which manifested itself in a profound fear of death. While other girls were falling in love for the first time, I was checking my body for any symptoms of a terminal illness. It was only when my mental problems started to have a physical impact on my body that I looked for outside help. I went through all kind of therapies and, in the end, I believe it was the restorative yoga that helped me most to let go of some of my fears and recognise that my anxiety was preventing me from living in the moment.

Although I still worry about not being a good enough mum or friend, I can now appreciate my life, give myself credit for what I have achieved and enjoy my very own kind of happiness.

Anxiety is a normal and necessary element of life. It is part of the fight-or-flight response, which prepares our body for action when in danger. Anxiety can become a problem when we get stuck in a constant fight-or-flight mode without there being a threat of real danger. This state of anxiety can be scary, exhausting and debilitating.

An estimated 275 million people suffer from anxiety disorders – around 3.5% of the global population – and women are slightly more affected than men. Countries with greater economic development and therefore, supposedly, better health and care resources, seem to have a higher incidence than other countries that are less economically developed.[2] The Covid pandemic led to a sharp rise in people affected by anxiety and depression and there is an increased urgency to strengthen mental health systems to deal with the increasing demand for support and help.[3]

My favourite 'therapy' besides yoga is dipping or swimming in cold water, regardless of the time of year. It is not suitable for everyone, so before you try it, consider the risks.[4] If you do go ahead, approach it slowly. Personally, I feel that the benefits significantly outweigh any risks.

I recently bought an old whisky barrel. We put it into our garden, filled it with cold water and much to the amusement of our neighbours, I sit in it for a couple of minutes every morning, doubling my out-breath to my in-breath. I close my eyes and breathe in through my nose, counting to 4 and exhale through my nose or mouth, counting to 8. This simple technique helps to slow my heartbeat, lowers my blood pressure and relaxes my muscles, while sitting in the ice-cold water.

The exposure to cold water makes me feel better because of the release of endorphins, feel-good hormones, and the decrease of cortisol, stress-inducing hormones. Also, cold water, even if it is just on your face, can activate the longest nerve in your body, the vagus nerve. This nerve connects your brain to many important organs, including the gut, heart and lungs. The vagus can influence your breathing (and vice versa) and heart rate, all of which can have a huge impact on your mental health.[5, 6]

However, if you feel on the edge of anxiety or shut down with fatigue and the cold-water therapy doesn't appeal to you, explore my other recommendations: yoga, controlled breathing and mindfulness.

The idea of yoga's positive impact on our mental health has been researched in many studies.[7, 8] Indeed, some argue that yoga should be clinically prescribed as a treatment for anxiety on the NHS.[9] While a lot of these trials are very promising, more research with larger groups of people will be needed to eventually convince the government and healthcare practitioners to clinically prescribe yoga.

A key player in managing anxiety is the breath. Deep and slow breathing can influence our mental and emotional state, and our thoughts and behaviours.[10]

I truly believe that when I can control my breath, I can control my random stream of thoughts and worries; something that yogis call the 'monkey-mind' (*Chitta Vritti*).[11]

The monkey-mind acts a bit like a hyperactive kid, flitting and jumping from thought to thought, especially at nighttime, from worry to worry, never concentrating on anything for very long. One way of dealing with this restless mind is to consciously relax your diaphragm (the muscle that helps you breathe) and to double your out-breath to your in-breath. This is easy to remember, even when you feel upset and anxious.

Try to incorporate doubling your out-breath to your in-breath, while performing simple yoga postures, such as the Cat and Cow Stretch (see p.54) or the Bridge Pose (see p.222).

Additionally, I like to use the Emotional Freedom Technique, EFT. It seems to work like acupuncture, but you use your own fingers to tap, rather than someone treating you with needles. EFT studies demonstrate its efficiency, with participants experiencing a significant decrease in anxiety and depression and an increase in happiness.[12]

Finally: mindfulness and meditation. It seems that meditating on a regular basis can be as effective as taking anti-depressants in improving symptoms of depression and anxiety, but without any unwanted side effects.[13]

Though, for some of us, meditation, the act of residing in a deep state of concentration, can be challenging and possibly not something you think you want to do when feeling anxious. Nevertheless, it is worth looking into and there are various ways to meditate. I recommend a visualisation based on images from nature, which can be soothing to your senses.

Explore some of the other mind-body experiences throughout this book (see Panic Attacks chapter, p.231 and Stress chapter, p.283), which can help you to live more in the present, instead of dwelling in the past or being anxious about the future. Furthermore, ditch multitasking! When you try to juggle multiple tasks at once, it can lead to a sense of feeling overwhelmed. Whereas when you take one step at a time and stay focused on one task only, you will be more productive, and feel less anxious.

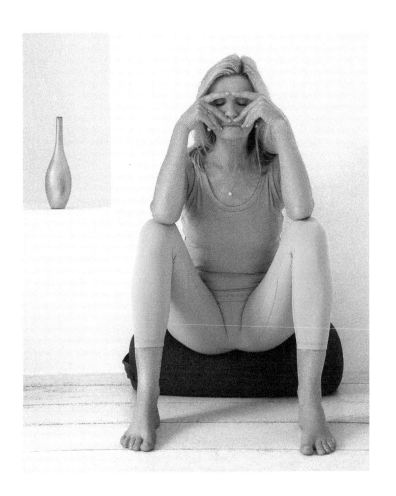

A key player in managing anxiety is the breath. Deep and slow breathing can influence our mental and emotional state, our thoughts and behaviours.

EXERCISES

OPTIONAL PROPS
Lavender and rose oil, blanket, block or cushion, chair

Legs-up-the-wall Pose
(Viparita Karani) and vagus nerve massage

You can do this pose anywhere, anytime, whenever you are feeling low or anxious or tired and exhausted. The true greatness of this pose is that it can teach you that from doing less, you can sometimes achieve more.

Caution: if you have glaucoma or a severe problem with your heart, be careful with any inversion - any upside-down position, where your head is positioned lower than your heart.

If you want to use the oil, have it ready and next to you. For added warmth, you may want a blanket to hand. Make sure that your belly is relaxed and not restricted by tight clothes. Use a little cushion if you need support for your head.

● **Sit down,** with your legs bent.

● **Lie back** and swing your legs, like a mermaid tail, up against the wall. Shuffle your bottom as close to the wall as possible. Support your lower back with a block or cushion if you like.

● **In a relaxed position,** adding some calming breaths will help to stop your anxious thoughts. Take a deep breath in through your nose and then release the breath out through your mouth, sighing. Research suggests that sighing can help you to return to a normal breathing pattern after experiencing an emotion such as anxiety or fear.[14] Repeat the deep in-breath and the audible out-breath again and again, until you feel a bit less anxious.

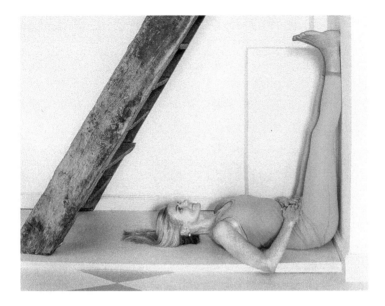

- **Double your out-breath** to your in-breath. Breathe in for a count of 4, then out for a count of 8. If this ratio is not right, reduce it to 3:6 or even 2:4. Repeat up to 10 times.

- **Then have a short break** before you start massaging your vagus nerve. Toning and stimulating this nerve can have a therapeutic effect when dealing with feelings of anxiety. If using, rub some drops of the lavender and rose oil into your palms, as if you are washing your hands with it, then cover your face with your hands and smell the soothing and calming effect of rose, clove, sage, patchouli and lavender.[15]

- **For the massage,** use both your middle fingers. To locate the vagus nerve, place your finger above the ear canal. Inside your ear, you can feel a ridge and above that a little hollow. Gently slide your fingers into the hollow and circle your fingers first clockwise, then anti-clockwise. No pressing or pulling, just gently massaging. You will probably want to sigh again – that's fine; just keep massaging and sighing, relaxing your jaw muscles. Eventually, after 1 minute, relax both your hands and remain in *Viparita Karani* for as long as you like.

Triangle Pose (Trikonasana)

The triangle can create *sama*, evenness. The full posture is a strong stretch that opens the sides of your body, increasing your breathing capacity. Unclench your teeth while holding the pose.

Caution: Be careful with this exercise if you have high blood pressure or a heart condition.

● **First come into the Mountain Pose,** *Tadasana* (see p.78). Bring your hands onto your hips, bend your legs and jump them silently 3-4ft apart. Turn your right foot out to 90 degrees and turn your left foot slightly inwards. Raise your right arm to shoulder height with your palm facing upwards. Bring the top of your left hand onto the back of your pelvis. Broaden your chest and lengthen your neck. Inhale and lengthen the spine, exhale and bend your body at your hip joint, stretching your right arm far out to the right side, as if someone is gently pulling you.

● **Then, place your right hand** just above or below your right knee. Encourage your chest to rotate up towards the ceiling. If this feels alright and your weight is evenly distributed between both your legs and feet, lift your left arm. There is no need to look up to your hand; rather keep your head neutral as that is much better for your neck.

● **Hold the triangle** for 2-6 breaths, then inhale and come back up to standing. Repeat on the other side.

MODIFICATION
If you feel a bit wobbly, practise the triangle with your back against a wall.

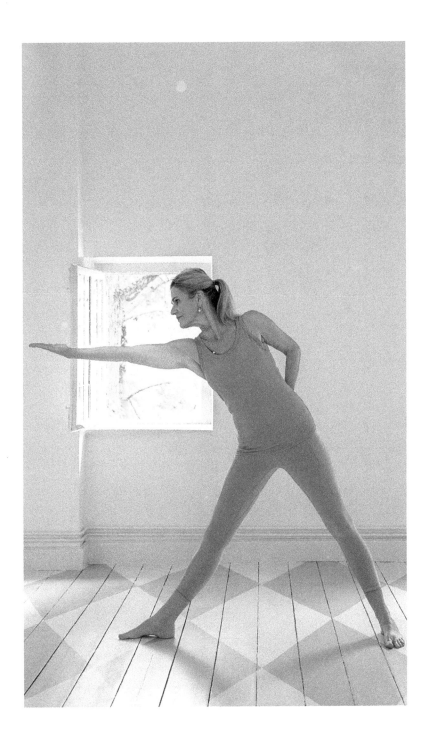

Emotional Freedom Technique
(EFT, Tapping)

The theory behind tapping is that all negative emotions are caused by a disruption in your body's energy system. By tapping certain energy points, while internalising positive statements, your brain and mindset can be reprogrammed. Tapping itself is comforting and relaxing, but in combination with a positive statement it can be even more powerful.

● **Take off your glasses** before you start the exercise. Sit comfortably on the edge of a chair, keeping your spine straight and your shoulders relaxed.

● **Identify the problem** you want to focus on and then create a positive statement, such as: 'Even though I feel anxious, I deeply and completely accept myself.' Of course, you can use any statement you like, but I suggest you try this one first and see how it works. It is important that you say this or your own statement with strength and conviction every time, as though you really believe in it and its power. Repeat the statement out loud and try to use all your fingers at each tapping point. Make sure that you tap with your fingertips, not your fingernails. The sound should be round and mellow as if you are drumming on a surface.

● **Repeat each statement 3 times**, moving in this descending order:

Eyebrows: 'Even though I feel anxious, I deeply and completely accept myself.'

Side of the eyes: 'Even though I feel anxious, I deeply and completely accept myself.'

Under the eyes: 'Even though I feel anxious, I deeply and completely accept myself.'

Under the nose: 'Even though I feel anxious, I deeply and completely accept myself.'

Chin: 'Even though I feel anxious, I deeply and completely accept myself.'

Collarbone: 'Even though I feel anxious, I deeply and completely accept myself.'

Upper chest: 'Even though I feel anxious, I deeply and completely accept myself.'

Top of the head: 'Even though I feel anxious, I deeply and completely accept myself.'

Repeat the whole sequence once more. You can extend the tapping further to your ribcage and the side of your hands.

● **When finished,** vigorously rub your hands and then cup them over your eyes for a moment. End with a big smile. As you smile, feel your jaw softening and a relaxed feeling spreading across your face, your entire head and down your shoulders.

Journey to a Safe Place
(Meditation)

It is evident that meditation can be an effective treatment for anxiety, and without any side effects.[16] Either ask someone to guide you through this visualisation or record the text on your phone and listen to it. For added warmth and comfort, you might want to snuggle into a blanket and sit on a block or a cushion with your back against a wall. If working with a partner, you can lean against each other back-to-back.

● **Close your eyes.** Bring awareness to your breathing and follow each in-breath and out-breath. If you are meditating with a partner, make sure that your lower backs are touching without leaving a gap. Feel the warmth and energy coming from them. Notice how you start synchronising your breaths.

● **Soon you will travel to a place** of your own imagination, a place where you can feel absolutely and utterly safe. A place you can return to whenever you need to. Stay with the first place that pops up in your mind when you hear the word *safe*. Try not to jump from place to place in the hope of finding something better.

● **Start exploring your place,** with your eyes still closed. Visualise where you are. Maybe somewhere in a beautiful countryside or somewhere in the city? Can you see yourself safely tucked away in your own bed or are you somewhere active at a beach or a lake?

● **Do you feel warm or cold?** Can you feel the sun, or wind and raindrops on your skin? Focus on these sensations while being calm, relaxed and feeling safe.

● **Now, bring awareness to your nose** and smell the scent at your place. Can you smell the scent of fresh bread or freshly cut grass? Or maybe the saltiness of the sea? Fresh washed linen or the delicious smell of your favourite dish? Whatever you can smell, stay with the scent for a moment.

● **Next, bring awareness to your ears.** What can you hear at your safe place? Maybe your favourite music? Or the chirping of birds, the far away noise of a boat or cars, laughter or silence? Whatever it is that you can hear, stay with it for a moment.

● **Eventually, bring back all your senses** to your own body and start to wiggle your fingers and your toes. Touch your lower teeth with the tip of your tongue. Listen to the sounds surrounding you. Open your eyes, look around you.

● **Lift both your arms,** stretch your upper body, hold your hands and bend from one side to the other before releasing your arms back down. Smile and, if you are working with a partner, turn around to see their smiling face.

● **Describe your safe place** to your partner and always remember, whatever happens, how sad or anxious you might feel, there is a safe place waiting for you.

This inner safe place is always accessible, and you can go and visit whenever you need to.

FURTHER TIPS

● **Smile!** Even a fake smile can stimulate the amygdala, the emotional centre of your brain.[17]

● **Voluntarily shaking** can be an effective way to manage your anxiety. Shaking it off is a valid response, a primitive mechanism to reset your muscle tension from a stuck state. I used to encourage my kids to shake, whenever they felt stressed or anxious, and it is a technique I often teach in my adult yoga classes. It is a good exercise to restore equilibrium in body and mind, and the self-induced 'electric shock' holds promising therapeutic value.[18]

● **Keep a mood diary.** Writing down what you are doing and how anxious you feel at different times of the day can help you notice what triggers feelings of anxiety. For some people it is obvious what makes them anxious, but for others it may not be so clear.

● **Set up 15 minutes** of 'worry time' each day. This should be the time when you can sit down, reflect over things that worry you and try to find solutions. Having this appointed time might help you to worry less throughout the day and night. When an anxious thought pops up, think 'I will set that aside for my worry time'.

● **Consider a talking therapy.** Choose your therapist wisely and try not to settle for the first available counsellor and therapy. In the UK, The British Association for Counselling and Psychotherapy (BACP) have a search function and provide tips on how to choose a therapist.

● **Get a weighted blanket** – the No. 1 household product in the USA – to help relieve stress and anxiety.[19] The pressure of the blanket is supposed to be calming. My clients love it.

● **Look into GABA** (Gamma-aminobutyric acid), a chemical messenger that we produce naturally in the body and that can play a key role in managing anxiety. Taking GABA supplements can help to lower feelings of anxiety and fear and support sleep.[20]

● **Alternatively investigate** *Ashwagandha*, a herb used in *Ayurveda*, the traditional medicine in India. It is best known for its anxiolytic (anti-anxiety) and stress-relieving effects.[21]

● **Some other helpful supplements for your nerves**, which you might want to try, are vitamin B9 and B12, inositol and omega-3 fatty acids, all necessary for the normal electrical functioning of your brain and nervous system.[22]

● **Be kind to yourself,** *Ahimsa*. Don't get worked up or annoyed with yourself for feeling anxious.

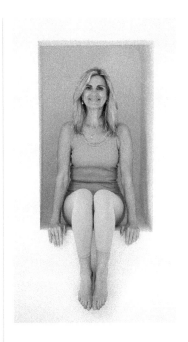

● **In the UK, you can call the NHS Helpline (111) or contact Anxiety UK,** www.anxietyuk.org.uk, a charity for those affected by anxiety and depression. As a member you can access workshops and support groups. The Samaritans also offer a safe place for you to talk. The response can take a couple of minutes, but the service is good and accessible. You can contact them via phone 116 123.

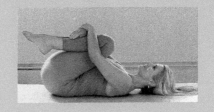

Back pain

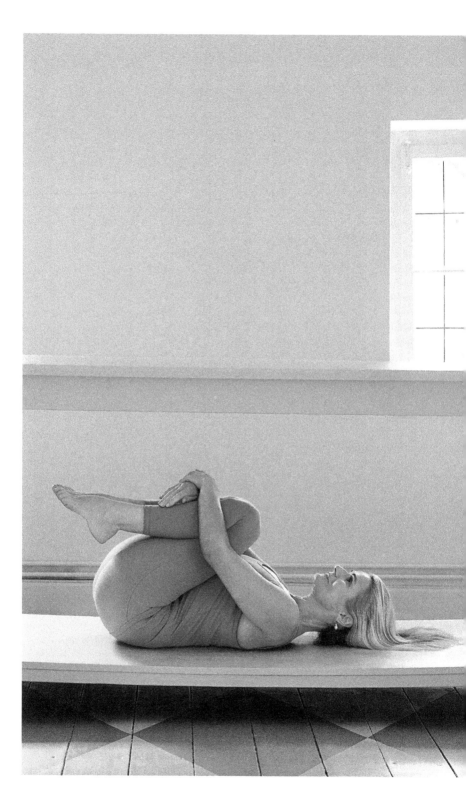

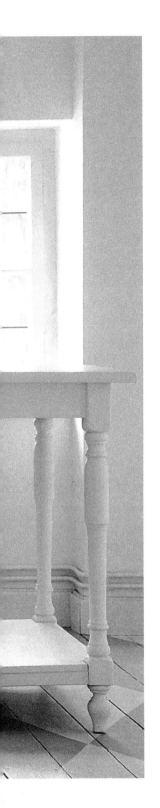

Back pain

> "Science is about to clone a human being, but it still can't cure the pain of a bad back?" [1]
>
> *Marni Jackson (Journalist)*

When one of my daughters got married, this joyful occasion triggered a few mixed memories for me. Seeing family members again after decades led to old issues re-emerging; difficulties I thought I had successfully put to bed suddenly haunted me again. My body reacted with severe lower-back pain, something I do not experience very often. It felt as if for years I had stored negative memories in my lower back and now there was no more space, my back seized up.

Thankfully, I recovered, but a lot of my yoga students continue to struggle to manage their back pain.

Whenever I teach, I ask what kind of physical problem they want me to address, and often the reply is: 'Please do something for the lower back – it hurts'.

An estimated 2.5 million people experience back pain every day in the UK and treating it costs the NHS more than a billion pounds a year. Lower back pain can affect all ages, from adolescents to the elderly, and is the major cause of sick leave in the adult working population.[2]

An endless number of ideas on how to cure back pain can be found online, including numerous home remedies for the best back pain relief. But, with all the medication and never-ending variations of sport and fitness programmes available, we still suffer from back pain. The truth is, finding a cure for back pain is not in the interest of those who profit from it. So, is back pain simply inevitable? One thing is for certain: there is not one single cure for all kinds of back pain. From a yogic perspective, back pain is commonly linked to posture, stress, muscle tightness and weakness – these are all issues that can be helped by doing the exercises in this chapter.[3]

However, be aware: the yoga poses that I recommend are not suitable for every type of back pain. People with specific spinal problems or slipped discs should seek specialist medical treatment. With any of the exercises, stop immediately if your symptoms worsen or you feel new or sharp pain. Use common sense and be aware that what you feel in your body trumps any recommendation from any yoga teacher.

Your spine has 24 moveable vertebrae. The lumbar spine (lower section) is more mobile than the thoracic spine (middle section), yet also carries more weight, making it the region of your spine most likely to cause pain. Furthermore, there are numerous muscles in your lower back. One group, the erector spinae, attaches to your spinal column at different points along your back, allowing you to bend from side to side and backwards. Toning and strengthening these muscles can help or even prevent back pain (see Osteoporosis chapter, p.217). On a spiritual level, the lumbar spine is connected to the so-called *Swadhisthana Chakra* (see p.329). This energy centre is the seat of your emotions, your sexual energy and creativity. This chakra can affect your reproductive system, bladder and lower back. I sincerely believe that we all tend to store negative memories and experiences of our childhood and early adolescence in this chakra. Letting go of these memories and emotions can help to release lower-back problems.

The middle part of your back is sturdier because the ribs are attached to the thoracic vertebrae, keeping this part of your spine more stable. Nonetheless, if you do experience pain in the middle of your spine, the cause is often due to poor posture, a sedentary lifestyle or incorrect use of equipment, e.g., spinning bikes with the handlebars set too high.

With any back problem, try to bring more awareness to your breath. You will be surprised how often back pain goes hand in hand with breathing problems. Slow and deep diaphragmatic breath (see p.112) can help to calm down an overactive stress response system, which will eventually help your muscles to relax, preventing painful muscle spasms.

I have included the 'Alexander Technique', which you might like to explore. Even though it is not a classic yoga exercise, this technique can be an effective way to manage long-term back and neck problems with no manipulation of your body involved. It is based on the relationship between your head, neck and back, and the aim of the exercise is to identify and change faulty postures and patterns (e.g., standing with your weight unevenly distributed) and to reduce your back pain by limiting muscle spasms, strengthening postural muscles and decompressing the spine.[4]

EXERCISES

OPTIONAL PROPS
Book or block, acupressure mat, blanket, eye pillow

Knees to Chest Pose
(Apanasana)

Although this is a very gentle exercise, stay tuned into your body and stop if you feel any discomfort.

● **Lie on your back** with your knees drawn up to your chest and place one hand on each knee. Relax your neck and face. Support your head with a book or block, if necessary.

● **Then, with your knees together, rotate them clockwise,** then anti-clockwise, massaging your lower back into the floor. Take your time and notice where you feel any comfort, discomfort or pain in your back.

● **If it feels doable, bring both your knees closer to your chest.** Then, gently push your knees away by straightening your arms. Keep your hands on your knees and your lower back on the floor.

● **Inhale deeply through your nose and pull your knees towards your chest**, lengthening your spine. Exhale slowly through your mouth and push your knees away, while pressing your lower back into the floor. Repeat up to 10 times, then practise it twice again throughout the day.

● **If your pain is located in the middle part of your spine,** modify this exercise slightly: exhale, pull the knees close to your chest and inhale, push the knees away.

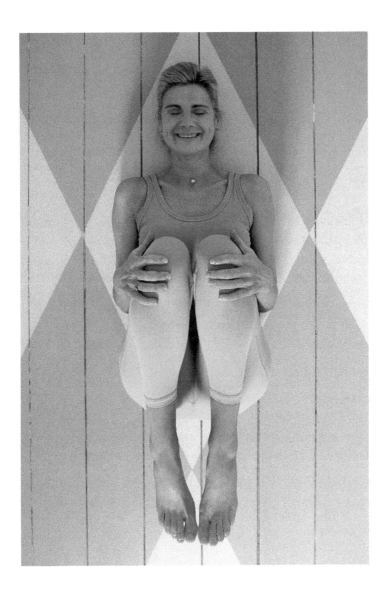

MODIFICATION

Use an acupressure mat (see p.333) underneath your back. The plastic needles can help to change your perception of pain. Despite the likely discomfort when first lying on this kind of pad, you will soon feel the benefits of the needle stimulation.[5] It's a bit like Marmite: either you love or hate it.

Cat and Cow Stretch
(Marjaryasana and Bitilasana)

This is a classic yoga exercise for back pain. If you do not like to be on your knees, perform the same spinal movements while seated.

Caution: Do not hold your breath if you have high blood pressure or glaucoma.

● **Start on all fours with your spine in a neutral position:** your knees directly beneath your hips and your hands below your shoulders with your thumbs pointing towards each other, thus taking the weight off your wrists.

● **Inhale:** lengthen and arch your spine. Exhale: round your spine. Start the movement from your hips and not from your head or shoulders.

● **Repeat** a couple of times.

● **Next time you round your spine,** come onto your fingertips, relaxing your head in-between your arms. Hold your breath while squeezing your buttocks, abdomen and lifting your pelvic floor.

● **Release your abdomen** and return to neutral, breathing in. Take time for a normal in- and out-breath without movement.

● **Breathe in,** arch your spine, lift your breastbone, hold your breath, before starting to round your spine. Breathe out, rounding your spine and retain the breath for a couple of seconds, elongating your lumbar spine. Release, come back to neutral and take a normal in- and out-breath before you start the next round.

● **Repeat at least 5 times.** When you feel comfortable, close your eyes and the whole exercise can become a moving meditation.

● **Once finished,** relax in Child's Pose (see p.241) either with your arms alongside your body and legs together, or with your knees wide apart and your arms extended. Keeping the knees together is better suited for very flexible yogis, whereas knees apart suits people who feel rather stiff.

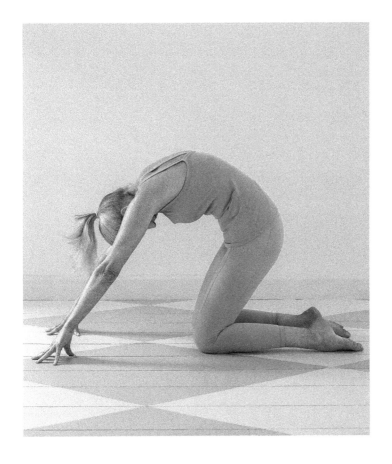

Happy Baby Pose (Ananda Balasana)

It is not the most graceful posture, but it can do wonders for your back. This playful pose puts the lower back into lumbar flexion, encouraging it to stretch out. Although beginner-friendly, someone with tight hips or a tight lower back can find it difficult to get into the position. If that sounds like you, practise the half baby, raising just 1 leg at a time.

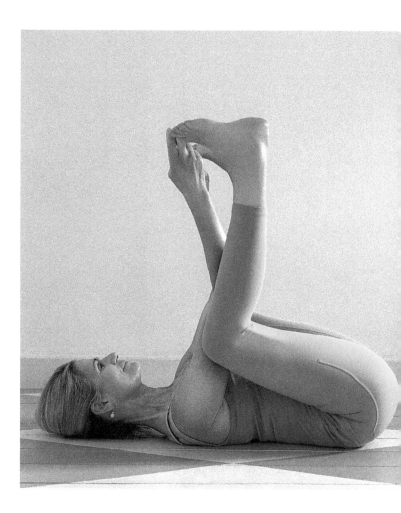

● **Lie on your back** and, if necessary, support your head with a book or a yoga block. Bend your knees towards your chest and belly. Now, lift your feet and grip the outsides, or grab your big toes with your middle and index fingers. Your arms are either touching the inside of your legs or they are in front of your lower legs. If you have difficulty holding your feet, then just hold the end of your trousers or your ankles.

● **Open your knees** wider than your torso and drop them towards your armpits. Bring each ankle directly over the knee, so that your shins are perpendicular, and your thighs are parallel to the floor. Gently push your feet up into your hands, as you pull your hands down to create some resistance. Ensure that your complete spine, including your tailbone, is down and flat on the floor.

● **Hold the posture for a couple of minutes,** using your out-breath to push away your tailbone and to soften your hips. Try not to drop your feet towards your bottom. Maybe gently roll from side to side, massaging the middle part of your spine.

● **When finished, roll over** to one side and slowly come out of the posture.

● **Try to practise this exercise** 3 times throughout the day. If you are feeling better, using an acupressure mat (see p.333) can speed up the healing process.

Corpse Pose Modification and Alexander Technique (Savasana)

In case you are not ready for any physical exercises yet, simply practise the Alexander Technique. Record the exercise and listen to it or ask a partner to guide you through it.

The Corpse Pose works even better for the lower back and neck in combination with the Alexander Technique. Evidence suggests that people who received one-to-one instruction in the Alexander Technique, along with regular yoga exercise, had reduced back pain and improved their condition after 1 year compared to those receiving standard care.[6]

● **Lie on your back** with your legs bent.

● **Place a block,** a couple of thin books, or a folded blanket under your head so that your chin is level with your forehead and your neck feels relaxed and at ease. Use an eye pillow if you like.

● **Position your feet reasonably close to your buttocks,** with your knees pointing towards the ceiling. Relax your arms, with your hands resting on your abdomen, without your fingers being interlaced.

● **First, focus on your breath** and notice your hands lifting with each in-breath and falling with each out-breath. There is nothing else you need to do; just keep observing your breath.

PAUSE

● **Now, you are ready to get engaged** into some Alexander Technique thinking. Let me make it clear that this exercise is not about relaxing or 'sinking' into the floor. Nor will there be any pushing, tilting or meditating, although the whole procedure will probably help to ease your mind.

● **Simply ask your whole back to lengthen!** Ask your spine to lengthen from the crown of your head down to your tailbone. While doing that, ask your neck muscles to release, which allows your spine to lengthen.

● **This way of thinking combines two key skills:** inhibition and direction. Inhibition is the message to stop doing, e.g., you don't push or stretch in order to lengthen the spine. The direction is through thought - you are simply sending an invitation to your muscles, without moving them.

● **Hence, you ask your neck muscles** to release so that your back can lengthen. Additionally, you ask your knees to point up towards the ceiling in order to help lengthen your back. And again: no pushing, pressing; just asking.

● **When you find that your mind wanders** during this procedure, just ask your back to lengthen and your neck muscles to release. This can happen once or twice or hundreds of times. You will always return to asking your back to lengthen.

● **If you do not get it the first time,** no worries, it will come with more practice. Perform this technique for at least 5 minutes 3 times every day for the next 6 weeks and you will feel an improvement and soon appreciate the impact on your neck and lower back.

FURTHER TIPS

● **Avoid the Boat Pose** (*Navasana*) in yoga classes. In this position, you balance on your sitting bones, with your legs lifted to form a V-shape. I have often seen people struggling with it, straining their back muscles rather than using their core.

● **Use a tennis ball** on the floor or against the wall to release the fascia (connective tissue) in your back. Roll the tennis ball into the parts of your spine that feel sore, stiff or painful.

● **When sitting at your desk**, try to sit up straight on your two sitting bones, not on your tailbone. So, roll onto the edge of your chair.

● **When lifting something heavy,** keep the object as close to your midline as possible to give you more stability and strength.

● **Push rather than pull.** Pushing, especially with your knees bent, uses more stomach and leg muscles and less of your back.

● **When sleeping,** try to avoid the embryo position because that tends to be the same position that you spend the whole day in, crouched over a desk. At least stretch out your legs while sleeping on your side. The best sleeping position for your lower back is probably lying on your back, but as a side-sleeper I know that this is not always feasible.

● **Stop wearing high heels.** They are sexy but deadly for your lower back. However, if you insist on opting for them, make sure that you stretch out your calf muscles, hamstrings and hip flexors with a fascia roll regularly.

● **Read *Back in Control*** by David Hanscom MD. It is a useful no-nonsense book for those suffering from chronic back pain.[7]

- **Use creams** that contain capsaicin or arnica, ibuprofen and menthol. These ingredients are soothing and safe.[8]

- **Invest in a good mattress.** When in doubt, opt for medium/firm memory foam or pocket spring. I found my ideal one after waking up pain-free in a hotel room and I copied the model number of that mattress.

Ditch your handbags and replace them with a stylish rucksack.

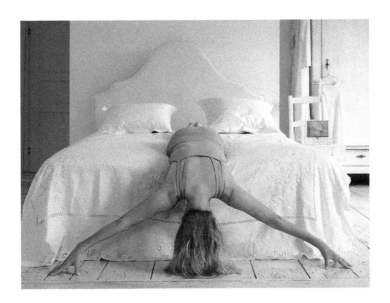

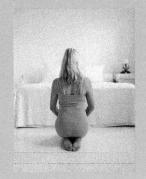

Constipation

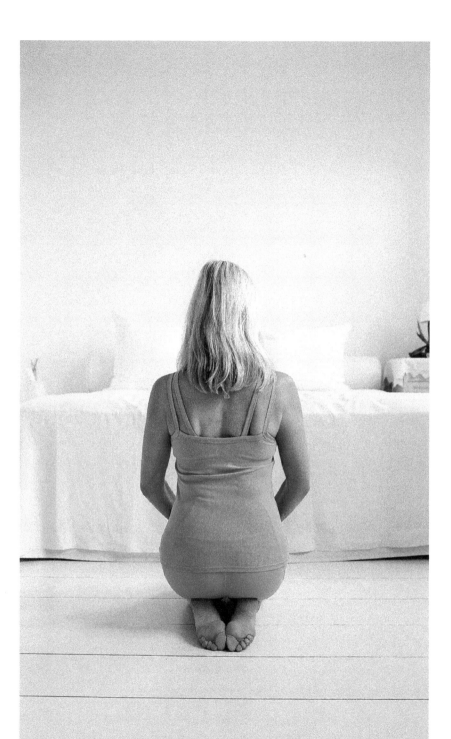

Constipation

"I wish that being famous helped prevent
me from being constipated." [1]

Marvin Gaye (Musician)

I envy people who wake up in the morning and everything
runs like clockwork. It doesn't seem to matter what
loo they use, whether they are alone or not, at home or
abroad, nothing disrupts their digestive routine. Everyone
has got to go when they have got to go, which seems simple
enough ... but what if you feel like a bloated duck, and you
can't get any relief as nothing is moving the way that it should?

Constipation is common and it can affect people of all ages;
even babies can suffer. Often the causes are linked to
insufficient bowel movement, inadequate physical activity or
genetics. Constipation seems more common among older
people and the use of laxatives is more likely in women. [2, 3]

Food, of course, can affect your digestion. Modern medicine
recommends drinking plenty of water and eating fibre-rich
foods – lots of fruit, nuts and vegetables – and avoiding all
those delicious things like warm white bread, fatty cheese
and sugar. I know, it is far easier said than done!

Ideally, I like to empty my bowels in the morning, as it makes me
feel more comfortable for the rest of the day. But that doesn't
work when there is not enough time, or the house is busy with
people coming and going. However, it is important to make

some peaceful time in your routine, in your own home, for your body. Try to train your bowels and go to the bathroom around the same time every day, ideally 30 minutes after eating.

Furthermore, I suggest that you reconsider your poo position. There is scientific proof that sitting on a white porcelain 'throne' is not healthy and could be the root cause of constipation and bowel problems, such as haemorrhoids, irritable bowel syndrome, even colon cancer.[4]

Did you know that squatting is physically the most efficient way to defecate, allowing your abdominal muscles to support the process of completely emptying your bowels? Squatting can relax your puborectalis muscle, straightening out your colon, therefore giving your faeces a direct route out – and all this without straining. So, how can you squat on your toilet? You don't need to be an acrobatic yogi or have specific skills to get into a good squatting position. Luckily, you also do not need to swap your loo for a hole in the ground. Try resting your feet on a couple of toilet rolls or a bathroom bin or invest in a 'Squatty Potty', a stool that raises your knees above your hips to put you into a squat-like position. I can guarantee you that it works!

How you breathe is important. Breathing in, holding your breath and pushing out your poo is not ideal. Instead, breathe out and engage your abdominals, widening your waist. Relax your pelvic floor muscles and anus muscles and literally breathe out your stool aided by gravity. Engaging your abdominals while sitting on the loo is simple: poke your index finger into your sides underneath your ribcage. Now push your fingers away with your muscles as you breathe out through your mouth. Can you feel your fingers being pushed away? This is what you want to do as you breathe out while letting go of your bodily waste.

A gentle do-it-yourself abdominal massage can be a superb way to loosen up. Research has shown that abdominal massage can relieve the symptoms of constipation more effectively than laxatives.[5] It only takes a few minutes of massaging in a circular motion to get things moving. The abdominal massage works by stimulating the peristalsis, the wave-like muscular contraction in your intestines that pushes everything through.

After the massage, practise a yoga twist to stretch and relax your muscles and intestines. Also, I like to recommend the Hero Pose, which does a really good job. Furthermore, look at the Flatulence chapter (see p.115) – some of the suggested yoga poses can also help with constipation.

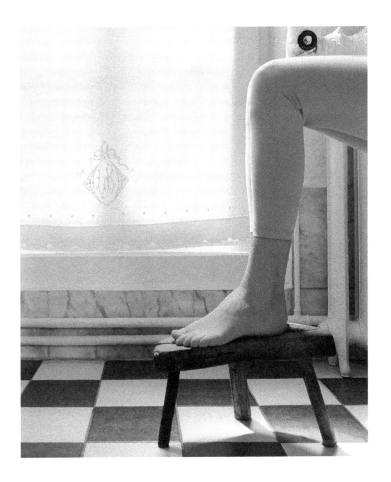

EXERCISES

Abdominal Self-massage

You can do this massage first thing in the morning, while still in bed. Ideally, use a few drops of fennel oil and rub your hands together, creating warmth and energy. The massage and the oil work best on your naked belly.[6] Do the stomach massage every morning for approximately 3 minutes. If it causes any pain or discomfort, lighten your pressure or stop.

Caution: Abdominal massage is not recommended if you are pregnant, if you have a hernia or if there is severe abdominal pain or discomfort, as it may indicate an issue that needs immediate medical attention.

● **Gently begin the massage** at the right lower side by your pelvis. You are going to use 1 hand only and massage in small circular motions, moving the tips of your fingers clockwise, and slowly working your way up the right side below your ribs, massaging there for at least 1 minute.

● **Now move your fingers over to the left side,** massaging below your left ribcage for another minute. Continue in small circular motions, slowly working your way down the left side before starting at the lower right side again. Practise a couple of rounds, slowly increasing the pressure of your fingers.

● **When finished,** shake out your hands and relax your arms.

Half-spinal Twist (Ardha Matsyendrasana)

This exercise should ideally be practised after the abdominal massage (see opposite page) and before breakfast. You can do a lying twist while still in bed.

● **Lie on your back** and bring your knees together onto your chest. Now place your arms out to the side at shoulder height with your palms up. Drop both your knees to the right side while keeping your left shoulder down. If your left shoulder cannot stay in position, bend your arm and place your hand onto your ribcage, relaxing your shoulder. Try to bring your knees as high up towards your arm as possible, because that will enhance the twist.

● **Hold the twist for several breaths,** gently squeezing your abdomen.

● **Then, bring first the top knee,** then both knees back onto your chest. Breathe in and with your next out-breath, drop your knees to the left side with your head remaining in a neutral position.

● **Repeat twice more** on both sides.

● **When finished,** drink a pint of warm water with a slice of lemon before you enjoy breakfast.

Hero Pose (Virasana)

After breakfast, practise the Hero Pose (see photo, p.64). This is the only yoga exercise I know that you can enjoy and perform well with a full tummy.

Caution: Do not practise this pose if you suffer from arthritis or have severe knee problems.

● **Kneel on the floor** and sit back on your heels. Feel your heels pressing into the sitting bones, separating the buttocks and stimulating your anal sphincter muscles.

● **If you cannot sit on your heels,** sit on a yoga brick with the small lateral side in-between your buttocks and sitting bones. This may not be very comfortable but will work and stimulate your muscles. To make it a bit more comfortable, you can support your knees with a cushion.

● **Place your hands onto your knees** with the palms facing down. Keep your spine straight and breathe normally while staying in the posture for 3 minutes.

● **If there is any discomfort in your thighs,** separate your knees a bit further. However, if you experience any sharp pain, come out of the posture immediately.

This is the only yoga pose I know that you can perform well with a full tummy.

FURTHER TIPS

- **Soak golden linseeds** in half a cup of water overnight. Then, first thing in the morning, drink the slimy juice, washing it down with a pint of warm water. It is gentle and efficient, and it works!

- **Go for the Kraut.** A helpful tip, and not just because I am German, is to eat a bit of Sauerkraut (fermented cabbage) in the evening. Sauerkraut contains probiotic bacteria that can help to improve your digestion and thereby reduce constipation.

- **Drink lots of still water.** Since constipation is related to dehydration of the colon, you need to make sure that you stay hydrated. This will soften your stool, making it easier to pass. If drinking more than 2 litres of water every day is not easy for you, try to drink the water with some lemon juice, rosemary or ginger to make it a bit more exciting.

- **If nothing else helps,** use glycerol suppositories to provide relief from serious constipation. It is best to add moisture to the suppository with a bit of tap water before you use it. Remember they are for rectal and short-term use only. I prefer suppositories to any other laxatives because they act locally and they don't cause cramping, which can be a concern with other laxatives.

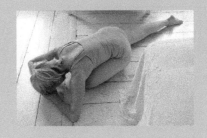

Eating
disorders

Yoga literally opened my heart, making me feel more forgiving towards myself and others.

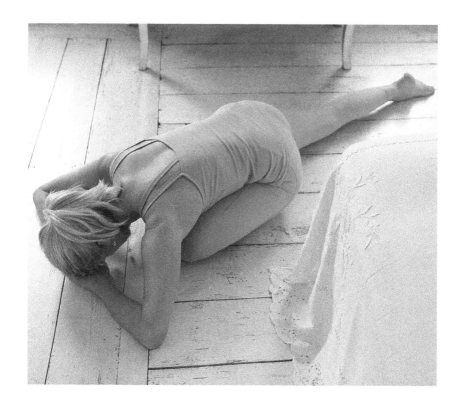

Eating disorders

"Every time I eat, I feel guilty." [1]

Freddie Flintoff
(TV Presenter and former England Cricket Captain)

We cannot survive without food. Yet, for some, eating can be a very sensitive issue and problem: either eating too little or too much. As a result, their relationship with food falls out of balance and turns into an obsession. However, unlike any alcohol or drug addiction, one cannot simply try to abstain from food. Therefore, curing eating disorders can be incredibly hard and re-establishing a good relationship with food can take a long time.

I was 15 years old when I became anorexic. I stopped eating substantial meals and instead loaded my plate with salad leaves, to cover up the fact that I was not eating properly. Nobody really knew anything about eating disorders at the time, so no one noticed me slowly fading away until a matter-of-fact paediatrician told my family that I was malnourished and that I should be force-fed.

Today, although there is a lot more information available, eating disorders continue to affect the lives of individuals and the people who love and want to help them. The number of hospital admissions in England with a diagnosis related to eating disorders has doubled within the last 10 years. In the UK, an estimated 1.25 million people have this illness and around 25% of those affected are male. Eating disorders have the highest mortality rate of any psychiatric disorder, from medical complications associated with the illness and suicide.[2, 3]

I survived. First the years of anorexia, then bulimia and binge eating, which lasted up until my mid-20s. It was a seesaw; I would eat nothing at all or literally everything. The overindulging then caused feelings of guilt, followed by starvation. A vicious circle.

Yoga did help me to eventually overcome and manage my eating disorders. In the beginning, simple yoga routines, which I watched and practised religiously every day on TV in the US, supported me with some stability, continuity and comfort. But then I used very strenuous yoga exercises to lose weight. I became obsessed with exercising just as much as I became obsessed with starving myself.

Thankfully, over time, I rediscovered the more nurturing aspects of yoga, including breathing techniques and mindfulness – exercises you can find in this chapter and the Anxiety chapter (see p.29) and Panic Attacks chapter (see p.231). Research shows that slow movements practised with full awareness gradually help to positively change self-perception, allowing you to become less self-critical, and I have found this to be true.[4]

Yoga literally opened my heart, making me feel more forgiving towards myself and others. Yogis call this contentment *Santosha*, appreciating yourself for who you are, how far you have come and all that you can look forward to.

Somehow, the slow healing process culminated in me becoming pregnant. Doctors had always told me that I was infertile because I never had any periods. Amenorrhea, the absence of menstruation, can often be a side effect of anorexia. However, affected women can still become pregnant and studies consistently report that fertility rates in women with a lifetime history of anorexia do not differ from women in the general population.[5, 6]

So, after years of struggling, I felt happy and light: my belly was full, with delicious food and new life, my baby daughter. This pregnancy marked the culmination of my recovery, representing a significant and final step in my healing process.

I sincerely hope that the following yoga exercises will help and encourage you to accept and love yourself for who you are: not perfect but very loveable.

Yoga remains my most enduring companion and is something that I will cherish forever.

EXERCISES

Mountain Pose and Self-hugging
(Tadasana)

Tadasana can help you to feel more grounded and the mindful hugging can bring reconciliation, healing and happiness. Furthermore, hugging releases oxytocin, the so-called 'love hormone', which can support the healing of eating disorders.[7]

- **Stand tall**, elongating your spine all the way up to the crown of your head.

- **Breathe in deeply through both your nostrils**, extending both arms out to the side, shoulder height, palms up.

- **Lift your breastbone and not just your chin**, gently arching your spine. Notice how the lengthening of your spine can already change how you feel within your body. Breathe out and cross your arms in front of you, literally embracing and giving yourself a lovely warm hug.

- **Breathe in and extend your arms out to the sides**, lifting your chest.

- **Breathe out, bend your legs slightly**, round your back, squeeze your bum and hug yourself again. Repeat this loving self-embrace and heart-opening exercise approximately 10 more times, alternating the top arm each time.

- **Remain in the last embrace** and then gently move your upper body from side to side as if you are rocking a baby in your arms.

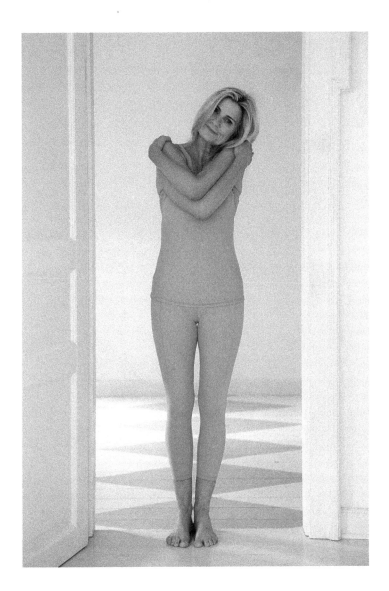

● **When finished,** relax your arms, straighten your legs and spine and stay in the Mountain Pose for a couple of breaths, with your eyes closed and a big smile on your face. Enjoy the moment, feeling grounded, lifted and in harmony with your body, breath and mind.

Dancer Pose (Natarajasana)

I consider this pose to be one of the most beautiful and elegant of all yoga poses. You can feel light and graceful, as you balance and bend forwards and backwards towards a solid wall. No matter what shape or weight you are, you will be able to perform this exercise. In case you struggle with your balance (lots of us do), stay close to the wall.

Caution: Do not perform the Dancer Pose if you suffer from acute back pain.

● **Stand, facing a wall,** positioning yourself approximately a foot away. Place your right hand against the wall and bend your left knee. Hold your ankle and bring your foot close to your bottom. If you cannot hold your foot or ankle, grab the end of your trousers to pull the leg up. The closer your knees are together, the more of a stretch you will feel.

● **Then, slowly crawl your right hand up the wall,** until your arm is fully extended. Press your right foot firmly into the ground as you push the left foot into your hand, up and away from you. Enjoy holding the stretch for a couple of breaths. Release and repeat on the other side.

● **Step an arm's length away from the wall** and lift your right arm towards the ceiling, with your thumb and index finger touching (*Chin Mudra*). Elongate your spine before you bend your left knee, bringing your foot close to your bottom. Try to hold the balance, without yet touching the wall.

● **Squeeze your inner thigh muscles** towards your midline as you hinge forwards from your hips. Touch the wall with just your middle finger while pushing your left foot into your hand, away from you.

● **Stay in the Dancer Pose for a couple of breaths,** saving your strength and energy to exit the pose with control. Slowly release first your arm, then your leg and foot, reconnecting both feet to the ground.

● **Relax for a couple of deep breaths** before you repeat the exercise with the other arm and opposite leg.

● **With more practice,** you may not need to use the wall. However, I still find it helps me to practise with more awareness, without worrying about my lack of balance.

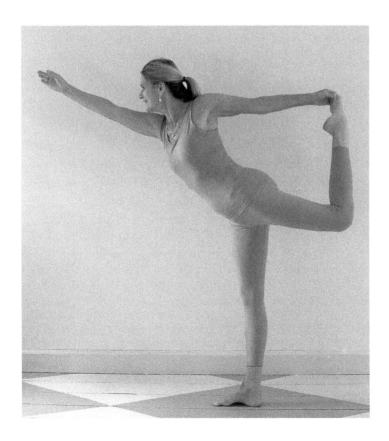

Heart Meditation

This heart-opening mindfulness exercise can help you to believe in yourself and others. Ideally, allow someone you trust to guide you through the meditation or record it on your phone, so that you can listen to it whenever you need to.

● **Sit on the edge of a chair** or lie on your back with your legs bent or stretched out. Support your head with a little cushion or block.

● **Focus on your breath for a couple of minutes** and bring awareness to your heart centre, the *Anahata Chakra* (see p.329). It is located below your sternum, your breastbone and often referred to as the 'Sea of Tranquillity' or seat of devotion and love. Place both of your hands onto your chest.

● **Close your eyes and visualise** a beautiful emerald green colour surrounding you, circling around your upper body. Green, the colour of nature and hope, can have a nurturing, harmonising effect on your body and mind, restoring depleted energy in your heart chakra.[8] Continue and watch the healing green light slowly entering your chest, filling your heart.

PAUSE

● **Now, seize the chance and visualise your own heart.** How does it look? Is it rather firm, like a fresh green pepper? Or soft, like a velvety cushion?

● **Is your heart shiny or matt, small or large?**

● **Stay curious and observe your own heart relaxing** and expanding.

● **Whenever your mind starts drifting away from your heart,** notice what takes your attention away. Acknowledge and identify the reason, but do not dwell on it. Instead, let go and return to observing your heart again. Repeat this process as often as necessary.

PAUSE

● **Now is a good time to let go of any negative feelings** and thoughts. Recall anyone or anything in your past that has hurt you. Whatever or whoever pops up first in your mind, stay with it or them. This can be about anything or anyone you know - perhaps a family member, your partner or a friend. What or whoever has hurt you, forgive and wish them well, let it go.

● **Then, visualise yourself as being strong** and in tune with your needs and instincts, knowing that you can make good decisions in your life and choose people who are kind and worthy of your love. Know that you can choose food that nourishes you and keeps you healthy.

● **Let go of any restrictions, feelings of guilt or regrets.**

● **Look forward to surrounding yourself with delicious food** and enjoying it with those you like and who support you.

● **Bring both your hands together** in front of your breastbone - *Namaste* - right in front of your heart and allow this hand gesture to connect you even further with your lovely inner self.

● **With your eyes still closed,** observe how the beautiful green light slowly recedes and finally disappears. Even though the green colour is fading away or changing into a red or pinkish colour, hold onto this positive and uplifting feeling that arises, once you open your heart.

● **Gently move onto your right side** and stay there for a while, before coming back up.

Victorious Breath (Ujjayi Breath)

This breathing technique is soothing, calming and audible. Because of its soft snoring sound, people call it 'Ocean Sound Breath' and others refer to it as the 'Darth Vader Breath'. You can practise *Ujjayi* on its own or during yoga postures.

Caution: If you have low blood pressure, slightly lengthen your in-breath to your out-breath. If you have high blood pressure, lengthen your out-breath to your in-breath and do not hold your breath.

● **Sit with one heel of your foot** pressing against your perineum. This is known as the Perfect Pose, *Siddhasana*. It stimulates the *Muladhara Chakra* (see p.329), the energy centre at the base of your spine. Imbalances of this chakra are often connected to eating disorders. Alternatively, sit on the edge of a chair with your spine straight.

● **Imagine that you are holding a mirror in front of you**, and you want to fog the mirror with your breath. Inhale through your nose, then exhale slowly through your open mouth, producing a long 'Haaaaaa' sound. Notice how the sound seems to narrow your throat a bit. Remember this feeling when you repeat the exercise, but with your mouth closed, breathing through your nostrils.

● **Once you have mastered the snoring sound** on your out-breath, try it on your in-breath as well. Imagine breathing in through a straw in your throat and this thought will help you to gently constrict your glottis, the opening between your vocal cords, which produces the characteristic sound of *Ujjayi*.

● **Practise every day for up to 3 minutes**, gradually increasing to 5 or 10 minutes over the next weeks and months. Try to be consistent and patient in your practice.

FURTHER TIPS

● **Nobody can fix you.** Though people can help you along the way, only you can make the changes you want to make. It is your actions that really count in your recovery and that will lead to freedom from your eating disorder.

● **Keep a record** of progress throughout your treatment and recovery. It is an effective way of keeping track of what you have achieved, when you doubt yourself or you are falling into the pattern of black-and-white thinking.

● **Practise** *Ahimsa,* which implies the end of violent words, thoughts or actions towards yourself or others. This then can increase your chances of falling in love again: with life and food.

● **Remember, you are not alone** and give people who love you the chance to help you. Or ask for advice when in need of help for yourself or someone else. Contact an eating disorder helpline. Phone 0808 801 0677 (England only) or email help@ beateatingdisorders.org.uk The helpline is open from 1pm-9pm during the week, and 5pm-9pm on weekends and bank holidays.

● **Seek therapy:** CBT (cognitive behavioural therapy) and IPT (interpersonal psychotherapy) can play a vital role in your ability to overcome an eating disorder.[9] Choose your therapist wisely. We tend to pick the right school, hairdresser and dentist very carefully, but may settle for the first available counsellor or therapist. The British Association for Counselling and Psychotherapy (BACP) website https://www.bacp. co.uk has a search function and provides tips on how to choose a therapist.

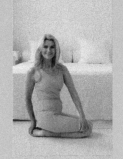

Fat belly

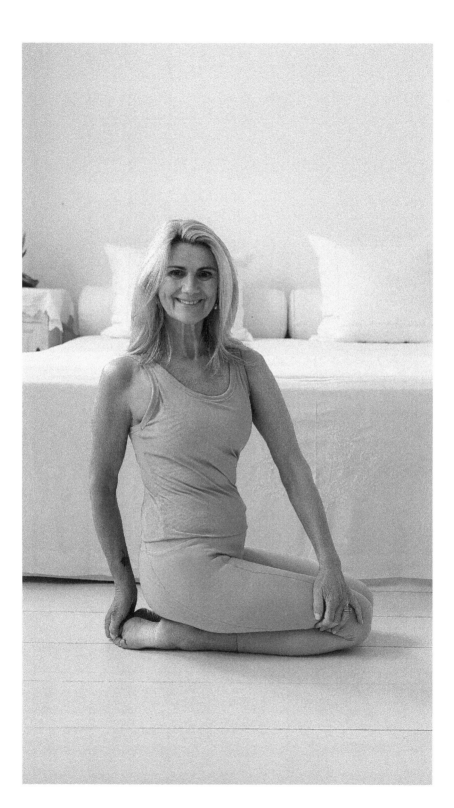

Fat belly

"My grandpa's family are all quite overweight
and he's got this big, rock-solid belly, which
I used to love to fall asleep on as a child." [1]

Daisy Lowe (Model)

Muffin-top, breadbasket, beer belly, spare tyre and food baby – there are a multitude of names to sugarcoat a fat belly, but I haven't yet met an adult who really loves their belly, me included. There are days I can make light of my belly, but admittedly I mostly try to hide it. My belly is often the first thing I look at or touch in the morning, checking if it is still there or if I can feel my hipbones.

When pregnant, I was very much in love with my belly. I felt empowered and proud of it. I gave birth to 3 beautiful children and somehow regained my figure every time, and I thought I would always be able to lose weight easily. But things changed when I entered menopause and developed not just 1 extra layer of belly fat but several and, to me, my body centre eventually turned into a wobbly meatball. My friends and husband tend to laugh about my concerns, but my belly messes with my mind, making me feel insecure.

The aim of this chapter is to encourage myself and others to embrace our bellies again. They are our powerhouses; never mind how fat they may be. The belly is the seat of our strength and willpower. It is where we first feel excitement or upset and where we can connect with our inner fire and the *Manipura Chakra* (see p.329).

There are 2 kinds of fat in our bellies: the subcutaneous fat, which is the soft layer of chub directly under our skin (harmless) and the visceral fat that forms around our organs (more dangerous). Visceral fat is strongly linked to serious health risks, including heart disease, cancer, kidney problems, type two diabetes and dementia.[2] Visceral fat is highly correlated to what you eat! So, all the exercise in the world will not help, unless you make some key dietary changes (see Weight Loss chapter, p.315 and Reflux chapter, p.253).

Some people tend to store more visceral fat than others. According to research, apple-shaped bodies can potentially conceal more health risks than pear-shaped bodies.[3] An apple-shaped body type has rather long limbs, culminating most fat in the middle. Whereas a pear-shaped body type has a smaller waist but larger hips and thighs. A person that is apple-shaped carries a higher chance of dying prematurely than any other body shape.[4]

We cannot change our genetic predisposition, but what we can change is our lifestyle, mindset, and the volume and types of exercise we do. The combination of all these can help to reduce a fat belly *and* boost our strength and confidence. Yoga, as well as pilates, can support you in toning and strengthening your abdominal muscles in a healthy and holistic way. However, do not expect a six-pack in 6 weeks. That would be unrealistic, and you will inevitably be doomed to fail.

In this chapter you will not find any belly crunches or sit-ups because they can potentially hurt your lower back or strain your neck when not done properly.

When working your abs, it is important to listen to your body, otherwise you may accidentally end up using your lower back and hip flexors instead.

I encourage you to feel and activate your deepest abdominal muscle, the *transversus abdominus* (TA), which is attached from your lower ribs to your pelvis and sits like a protective corset around your middle.

Plan on doing daily repetitions (slowly increasing the number) of my recommended exercises and your body will begin to respond with a stronger, toned core and more ease in your movements, resulting in a more powerful and confident version of you.

Another helpful tool in toning your belly is the breath. Not the usual in- and out-breath but controlled breathing, like *Kapalbhati,* the Skull Shining Breath. It is also a cleansing exercise, a *Kriya,* and it consists of short and powerful exhales and passive inhales through both your nostrils. It can strengthen and tone your diaphragm and stomach, thus helping to reduce the circumference of your waist.[5] Furthermore, reconnect with your centre and practise the Love Your Belly Breath (see p.262).

EXERCISES

Skull Shining Breath
(Kapalbhati)

Sometimes known as 'The flying bogey', for reasons that will become clear, this breathing technique can literally blow your brain, boost your oxygen supply and tone your abdominal muscles.

Caution: Do not practise *Kapalbhati* if you are pregnant, or if you have a respiratory infection, high blood pressure, any cardiac issues or suffer from panic attacks, epilepsy or diabetes.

● **Blow your nose,** before you start this exercise, to enhance the effectiveness and comfort.

● **Sit comfortably on the floor,** or on the edge of a chair or bed, with your feet below your knees. Connect with your sitting bones, which can help you to straighten your spine. Relax your hands either on your thighs (palms up) or bring them into a diamond shape on your lower abdomen, with your thumbs pointing towards your navel.

● **Breathe in** and feel how your belly expands.

● **Breathe out** and feel a gentle contraction as your belly moves towards your spine. Follow your breath for a short time, then imagine that you want to blow out a candle by breathing out forcefully through both your nostrils. Try to keep your mouth shut throughout the exercise. While breathing out vigorously, your belly, and the little jugular notch in your neck, will move in and out but nothing else should move.

● **Do not move your shoulders or head;** simply focus on breathing out through both your nostrils. Do not think about breathing in, because that will happen automatically.

● **Start slowly, gradually picking up speed:** out, out, out. Eventually finish with a deep in-breath and hold your breath for a couple of seconds before you slowly breathe out again. This time through your mouth.

● **Practise a couple of short rounds first** and, with time, you will be able to do up to 25 or perhaps even 50 out-breaths. The best time to perform *Kapalbhati* is in the morning before breakfast. If you struggle, do not worry – rest and start again.

● **If you feel lightheaded after this exercise,** no worries. It is normal and this feeling will usually lessen with time and practice.

Toe Taps

First, try to find your *transversus abdominus* - TA muscle. Lie on your back and bend your legs with your knees apart. Bring your hands into a diamond shape on your lower abdomen below your navel. Now laugh or cough, whilst holding your abdomen. Can you feel a muscle as you cough? This is the TA muscle, the one you want to work.

Now, you are set up for the Toe Taps exercise. Precision is key with this exercise if you want to successfully tone your belly and not accidentally strain your back.

● **Lie on your back** and bring your hands into a diamond shape on your lower abdomen, with your thumbs pointing towards your navel.

● **Lift your bent legs** and create a right angle (90 degrees) with your thighs vertical and your lower legs parallel to the ground. Flex your feet, keeping your heels in line with your knees and your knees in line with your hips.

● **Throughout the exercise** try to keep your TA muscle engaged but relax your shoulders and face. Ideally, breathe in and out through your nose; alternatively breathe out through pursed lips.

● **Tap** first your right set of toes on the ground, then your left.

● **In-between return to the starting position,** creating the right angle with both your legs bent, your knees in line with your hips and your feet flexed.

● **Breathe in as you hold the angle,** breathe out as you tap first one foot, then the other. Work slowly and with precision with your knees staying in line with your hips. As you go faster, your breathing can change into *Kapalbhati* (see p.92).

● **First practise 10 to 20 toe taps,** then increase up to 30 or 50 times each side.

● **Practise 2 rounds,** ideally one after the other, every day.

● **There can be a third round** where both legs are at a right angle and you tap the floor with both feet at the same time, then bring them back up to the starting position.

● **Whenever you feel** that you are bringing your knees closer towards your chest, or your lower back is arching, stop immediately. Have a little rest, hug your knees into your chest and start again.

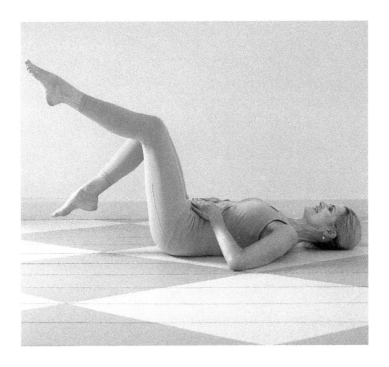

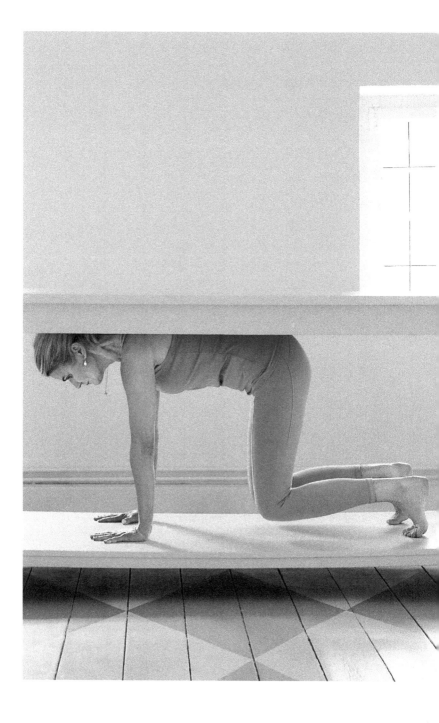

Tabletop Lift (Bharmanasana)

This exercise is simple and so effective.

Make sure that your head remains above or slightly in front of your hands to work your abdominal muscles. If you move your head back, you will be working your thighs instead of your belly. Keep your arms straight - no hyperextension - and do not drop your head.

● **Come onto all fours,** with your spine in a neutral position. Make sure your knees are in line with your hips, and your hands are directly beneath your shoulders. Spread your fingers apart, with the middle finger pointing straight forward and your thumbs pointing towards each other, to take the pressure off your wrists.

● **Lengthen your neck** so that your head is slightly in front of your hands and the back of your head stays in line with your spine. Press the heels of your hands firmly into the floor to flatten your shoulder blades into your back.

● **Curl your toes under** and lift both your knees a couple of inches off the floor. Hold the pose and breathe out forcefully through your nose or through pursed lips for around 20 breaths.

● **Relax for a moment** and repeat once more if you like.

● **Relax in Child's Pose** (see p.241) when you have finished.

Meditation on Your Inner Sun

Ideally, ask someone to guide you through this exercise or record the meditation on your phone.

Consider using some lemon/lemongrass and fennel oil, which when inhaled, diffused or rubbed, may help to reduce cravings, boost your energy levels and promote weight loss.[6]

Caution: Do not put the oil directly onto your face.

● **Lie down on your back** and relax. Close your eyes if you like. Bring awareness to your centre. Place both hands on your tummy, fingertips touching. Inhale and feel your belly expanding; exhale and feel your belly contracting.

● **Stay focused on your belly,** the seat of the *Manipura Chakra* (see p.329), which is one of the 7 main chakras throughout your body. The element of this chakra is fire, and it is the seat of your strength, vitality, ego, willpower and stamina. The *Manipura Chakra* can influence your digestive system, gall bladder, pancreas, adrenals and liver.

● **Now, visualise golden *Prana*,** energy, slowly flowing into your centre, filling your belly with a beautiful golden colour.

● **Imagine that your belly is just like the sun:** golden and warm. Your inner sun is radiating light and heat - energy - which makes it possible for you to exist and to succeed. And just like the earth needs the heat of the sun, your body relies on an active and radiating energy centre, the *Manipura Chakra.*

● **Direct your breath into your golden centre** and connect even deeper with your strength, feeding the warmth, the energy within you.

● **Your powerful golden sun** spins evenly, radiating its power to all the other parts and energy centres within your body.

● **You might notice your mind drifting away** from your sun. Do not worry, that is what minds do. Just gently bring back your attention to your belly, the golden shiny ball at the centre of your being. The shifting of your mind and you refocusing on your belly can happen once or twice, or hundreds of times. It doesn't matter; just be aware of this process and keep returning to the image of your golden centre.

● **Welcome and nourish your golden sun** and continue to imagine it spinning in harmony with all the other chakras within your body, below and above your belly.

PAUSE

● **Slowly, allow the image of the sun to fade,** but hold onto this feeling of strength and confidence. Release your hands, open your eyes and come up into sitting. If you're using it, sprinkle a few drops of the oil onto your hands. Then cup your hands in front of your face, inhaling this lovely fresh, energising blend.

● **End by bringing your hands together in front of your heart** into *Namaste*, turn your fingertips down towards your abdomen and then up again. Briefly bow your head towards your heart, smile and relax your hands.

FURTHER TIPS

● **Reduce sugar.** A sugar detox can be one of the most efficient ways to tackle the fat around your abdomen. When eating too much sugar, your body releases insulin to bring the blood sugar level back into balance. But insulin can hinder the burning of fat stored in your belly.

● **Look into a medication called metformin.** There can be beneficial effects of metformin on visceral fat reduction.[7]

● **Investigate the amino acid L-arginine,** which you can find in high-protein foods, such as peanuts. A pilot study showed some evidence that L-arginine has weight loss promoting powers and was found useful in treating central or visceral obesity.[8]

● **Try to manage stress** because the stress hormone cortisol will increase your appetite and that will show around your abdomen and waistline. See Stress chapter, p.283.

● **Go back in time** and get a Hula Hoop – yes, the exercise ring, not the snack! It's fun and can make you fall in love with your belly, while playfully burning off calories.

● **Try to ignore** unrealistic societal expectations and relax your attitude towards your belly (e.g., when you are posing for photos).

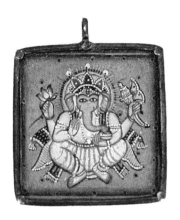

Take *Ganesha*, the
Elephant God, as an
example. Just looking
at his big fat belly
makes me happy.

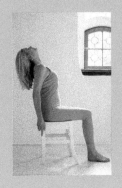

Fibromyalgia

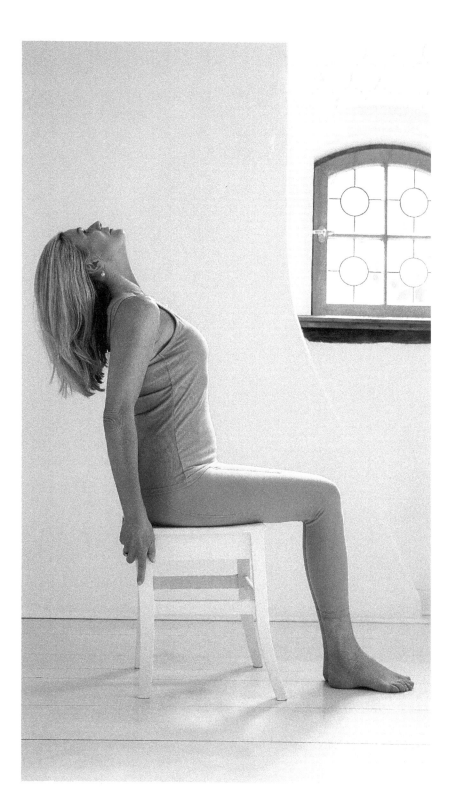

Fibromyalgia

*"I get so irritated with people who don't
believe fibromyalgia is real."* [1]

Lady Gaga *(Singer and Songwriter)*

For years, I wondered what was wrong with me because everything seemed to hurt: my neck, chest, shoulders, elbows, hips, knees and toes. I felt tired, lacked energy and found it hard to concentrate on menial tasks such as reading a book or following simple instructions. Whenever I mentioned this to my GP, I was told it was probably related to the menopause, and that I shouldn't worry. So, I started taking HRT, which seemed to help in the beginning, but soon the pain returned, worse than before. I decided to pay for a consultation with a rheumatologist. It was then that I heard about fibromyalgia for the first time and suddenly it all made sense.

Fibromyalgia, chronic pain, seems to be related to abnormal levels of certain brain chemicals and changes in the way the body's central nervous system processes pain messages. In some cases, the condition can be triggered by physically or emotionally stressful events. The illness can occur in people of any age, including children, but typically develops between the age of 30-50. It affects way more women than men and seems to be more common in people with joint hypermobility, something you often see in yoga teachers.[2]

Fibromyalgia is a relatively unspecified illness and for a long time doctors suspected that this chronic pain might be predominantly psychological – unfortunately, there are still those who consider people affected as hypochondriacs. However, in the UK, the Department for Work and Pensions (DWP) now recognises fibromyalgia as a real and potentially disabling condition of unknown cause.[3] As yet, there are no specific tests to confirm that someone has this chronic pain disease and so recognition and diagnosis can take a long time.

Getting enough sleep is essential when coping with fibromyalgia and a non-restorative sleep, waking up in the morning without feeling rested, can be one of the strongest predictors for developing chronic pain.[4]

So, what can you do when you think you have fibromyalgia? First, accept that the pain you feel is real and that it is not just in your head! You do not have to convince anyone that it exists. Then, find a rheumatologist who is familiar with the illness and insist on a referral from your GP. Consider taking the medication they might prescribe, often tricyclic antidepressants.[5] I was prescribed a low dose of nortriptyline and it helped. My pain perception changed, and it improved my sleep. I can cope without it now, but it gives me a sense of security knowing that there is something that works if I need it.

Even though I took the medication, I cannot stress enough how important it is for me to practise yoga every day as it helps me to calm my overactive nervous system (see Stress chapter, p.283). I find that the exercises in this chapter,

Pawanmuktasana, are ideal to loosen my stiff and painful joints. The *Pawanmuktasana* exercises are divided into different groups. In this chapter we focus on Part I, the anti-rheumatic group.[6, 7]

I often feel tension in my upper back, shoulders and neck. This is where 10 of the 18 typically tender points of fibromyalgia are located and I recommend gentle, but invigorating backbends, such as the Sphinx Pose, which can lengthen and strengthen your spine and neck.

Besides yoga, I swear by cold water swimming (see p.32), deep tissue massages and my acupressure mat (see p.333). Using the mat while performing some of the exercises considerably reduces pain, especially in combination with a slow diaphragmatic breath.[8, 9, 10]

I cannot stress enough how important it is for me to practise yoga every day as it helps me to calm my overactive nervous system.

EXERCISES

Anti-rheumatic Group
(Pawanmuktasana Part I)

Small joint movements can stimulate the flow of synovial fluid
at friction points where your tendons pass over bones in your
shoulders, fingers, hips and knees. The following exercises are
not challenging and can be practised even by a yoga novice.
Aim to perform the whole sequence 3 times per day. You can
practise sitting on a floor or on the edge of a chair with your
legs bent. If tired, rest in-between the poses and remember
that less is more. Learn to accept, adapt and accommodate.

SHOULDERS AND UPPER BACK

● **Sit upright** using one or two yoga blocks if you wish, with
your legs extended out in front of you. Bend your legs slightly
if you have tight hamstrings. Flexing your feet will help to keep
your spine straight. Relax your arms by your side.

● **Breathe in and lift your shoulders up to your ears.** Breathe
out, roll your shoulder blades back and down. Repeat
10 times.

● **Then, practise the shoulder rolls the other way around:**
squeeze your shoulder blades together, lift them, move them
forwards and down.

SHOULDERS AND NECK

● **Relax your arms on your thighs**. Look straightforward with your shoulders pulled back and down. Tuck your chin in, to resemble a double chin. Hold this position, but not your breath, for 5 seconds, breathing smoothly. Perform up to 10 times. Relax and repeat.

FEET AND ANKLES

● **Relax your neck and shoulders** and place your hands beside you, with your fingertips pointing forwards, and slightly behind your buttocks. Now flex and point your feet 10 times – inhale as you flex and exhale as you point.

● **Repeat,** but this time exhale as you flex your feet and inhale as you point your feet.

● **Slowly lift and rotate your right foot** 10 times clockwise and 10 times anti-clockwise. Repeat with your left foot. Keep your spine straight as you lift and rotate your ankle.

● **Finish by relaxing your legs and feet,** and come into an easy cross-legged seated position.

Remember that less is more.
Learn to accept, adapt
and accommodate.

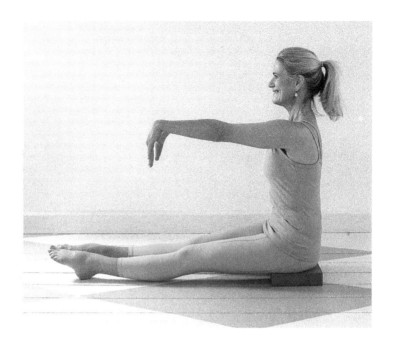

SHOULDERS AND ARMS

● **Extend your arms out in front of you** at shoulder level. Inhale, keep your arms straight and bend your hands backwards from the wrists so that your fingers are pointing towards the ceiling. Then, exhale and bend the hands forwards from the wrists so that the fingers are pointing towards the floor. Repeat up to 10 times.

● **Relax then extend your arms out in front of you** and rotate both your wrists (not your arms) 10 times clockwise and anti-clockwise.

● **Finish by shaking out your hands.**

Sphinx Pose (Salamba Bhujangasana)

This pose can gently stretch the back, chest and abdominal muscles and that can help to ease some stiffness and pain.

Caution: The Sphinx Pose is not recommended if you are pregnant. If you experience any sharp pain or a pinch while being in the Sphinx, come out of the pose immediately.

● **Lie on your tummy.** Bring your elbows underneath your shoulders, keeping them parallel to each other. Gently press your elbows into the ground to enable you to lift your breast-bone, while elongating your spine. Keep your chin parallel to the floor. Your legs should be straight, in line with your buttocks. Try to hold the exercise for 10 deep diaphragmatic breaths.

● **If you feel any discomfort**, press your pubic bone into the floor and squeeze your glutes to decompress your lower spine.

● **You might want to turn your head** to the right, back to centre and then to the left. Move your head as you exhale. Lengthen your neck as you inhale. Repeat 3 more times.

● **To end, bring your elbows out** to each side and lower your head, resting your forehead on your hands. Wiggle your hips a bit from side to side before you push yourself back up.

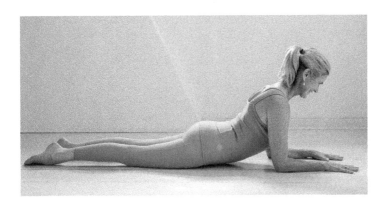

Supported Relaxation Pose
(Savasana)

In this relaxation pose, you will meet your new best friend: the diaphragmatic breath. When pain seems overwhelming, use your breath to ease your pain perception and for comfort.

● **Lie down and bend your legs,** without your knees falling towards each other. You might want to place a bolster underneath your knees and support your arms and head with a block or small cushion. Use a blanket if you feel cold and massage a bit of basil oil onto your wrists if you like. Or try lying on an acupressure mat – the stimulation from the plastic needles can help to decrease your sensitivity to pain. Despite the possible discomfort when first lying on the mat, you will soon feel the benefits. Either you will love or hate it. I love it!

● **Once you are settled into the pose**, simply breathe in and out through your nose. The breath will find its own pace, and even if you believe the speed to be too fast or too slow, you don't need to control it, just breathe.

● **Move your attention to your abdomen.** Feel how your belly lifts as you inhale and flattens as you exhale. Place your hands onto your belly to physically feel the rise and fall.

● **As you slowly inhale**, soften the muscles of your lower back and abdomen and allow your back to rise and expand. It may feel as if your lower back is being stretched by your deep in-breath.

● **Repeat the long exhale and inhale a couple of times**, until you become accustomed to the feeling of deep inhalation.

● **Eventually, return to your normal breath** and allow yourself to stay in the relaxation pose for as long as you like.

FURTHER TIPS

● **Forget painkillers,** such as ibuprofen and naproxen. They are generally not very effective in easing the pain of fibromyalgia. But what can help is carbamazepine, a medication normally prescribed for people with epilepsy.[11] Please discuss with your GP.

● **Nose drops** containing the hormone oxytocin seem to help with chronic deep tissue pain.[12]

● **Try cannabis products short-term and basil oil,** which are natural and can be useful for the treatment of fibromyalgia.[13, 14]

● **If you opt for injections** with a local anaesthetic directly into tender points, make sure that you mark the points yourself, so that the doctor can see where you feel the pain. You may need to repeat the procedure a couple of times for maximum effect.

● **Try cognitive behavioural therapy (CBT)** or a talking therapy. It can improve your ability to cope with pain and a low mood.

● **Find your *Sangha*,** your community of yoga teachers, practitioners and other people dealing with fibromyalgia. Sharing information with one another will make you feel less alone or misunderstood.

● **Fibromyalgia Action UK** is a charity that offers information and support to people with fibromyalgia. The charity's helpline is 0300 999 3333 in the UK. https://www.fmauk.org/contactsmenu.

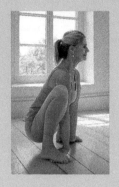

Flatulence

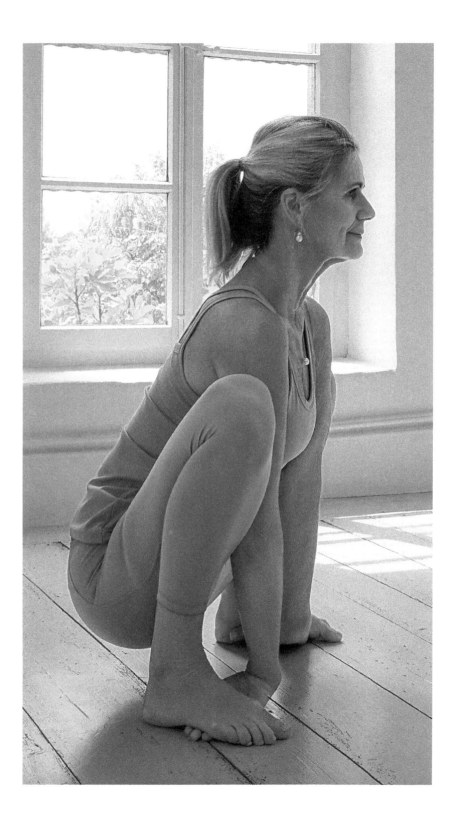

Flatulence

"A happy fart never comes
from a miserable ass." [1]

Martin Luther (Priest)

must admit that the older I become, the more I enjoy farting. I know it is a slightly awkward thing to say, but an unrestrained toot can feel good, even cathartic at times. There is something liberating about it. Gone are the days of desperately squeezing bum cheeks together to carefully release only the slightest bit of wind from a bloated gut, hoping for no sound to be made. How incredibly repressive.

Yet, I accept that farting is not very sexy and that it is sometimes embarrassing. I also know that it can annoy loved ones. My family set up an annual challenge – instead of 'Dry January', we practise 'Fart-Free February'. The aim is not to break wind in front of each other for a whole month. Which is harder than you might think …

Everyone farts: the King, the Pope and the Dalai Lama. The average amount is between 10-15 times per day. Excessive (more than 20) or smelly wind can be caused when you swallow air or eat food that is difficult to digest. The usual culprits are meat, onions, garlic, leek, dairy, sprouts, broccoli, cabbage, raisins and beans. If you want to reduce farting, then avoid these foods or eat only small meal portions, and don't gulp. Stop chewing gum or using artificial sweetener. Furthermore, stay away from carbonated drinks and beer. The best alcohol to drink is gin, vodka and tequila on the rocks. If you are a wine lover, go for red.

Farting in yoga classes is quite common. As a yoga teacher you tend to ignore it. Increased farting can happen during *Pawanmuktasana* Part II and Part III, the digestive and abdominal group of exercises, that can help to get rid of excessive air and eliminate energy blockages in the abdominal energy centre, the *Manipura Chakra* (see p.329).[2]

There are several useful and practical yoga exercises to help you release trapped wind. You can practise them regularly or strategically before important meetings or social gatherings. The exercises that I recommend are to release wind, not to prevent it because farting is normal and it is healthier than suffering in silence from painful trapped gas in your intestines.

I must admit that the older I become, the more I enjoy farting. An unrestrained toot can feel good, even cathartic at times.

Happy Baby Pose
(Ananda Balasana)

This is an easy and relaxing pose (see photo, p.56) that helps to release trapped gas. It is the posture to do before going out on a first date or any other important occasion where you do not want to break wind in front of strangers.

● **Lie on your back** and, if necessary, support your head with a book or a yoga block. Bend your knees towards your chest and belly. Stay there for a moment, pressing your thighs against your abdomen.

● **Now, lift and grip the outsides of your feet** or grab your big toes with your thumb and middle and index finger. Your arms should be either touching the inside of your legs or be in front of your lower legs. If you have difficulty holding your feet, hold the end of your trousers.

● **Open your knees wider than your torso** and drop them towards your armpits. Bring each ankle directly over the knee, with your shins perpendicular, and thighs parallel to the floor.

● **Gently push your feet up into your hands,** as you pull your hands down to create some resistance. Relax the muscles around your anus and try to widen your legs a little bit more. Hold the posture for a couple of minutes before releasing your legs again. Repeat.

Wind-Releasing Pose (Vayu Nishkasana)

This pose (see photo, p.116) can help to alleviate bloating and gas by massaging and stimulating your abdominal organs. It is a classic pose for relieving flatulence.

Caution: Do not practise this if you suffer from knee or back problems. Be careful if you have very high or low blood pressure. Keep your eyes open throughout the exercise and take off any rings.

● **Come into a deep squat** with your feet more than hip-width apart. You may want to use a block or book underneath your heels. Your toes and knees should be slightly pointing outwards. Touch the insteps of your feet, placing your fingers under the soles. Your upper arms should be gently pressing against the inside of your knees.

● **Inhale,** lifting your chest and head, and lengthening your spine.

● **Exhale,** raising your bottom, straightening both legs and relaxing your head in front of your knees. Do not worry if your legs are not straight. Take a long in- and out-breath. Remember to inhale in the squatting position and to exhale in the raised position.

● **Repeat up to 5 rounds,** then relax standing in a forward bend with your arms dangling. Very slowly come up to standing, counting to 33 as you curl up each vertebra one by one. Do not touch your legs as you come up as this encourages your legs to relax – it is more effective to engage your leg muscles and to avoid any strain on your lower back.

Rocking and Rolling
(Jhulana Lurhakanasana)

Another wind-releasing pose, this one massages the muscles along your spine and it can reduce the build-up of gas in your digestive system. The best time to practise is early in the morning to wake up your body and your digestive system.

Caution: Be careful not to hit your head on the floor when rolling backwards. Do not perform this exercise if you have any serious back and neck problems.

● **Lie down and bring both your knees onto your chest.** Place your hands behind the backs of your knees. Tuck your chin in and gently swing your legs over towards your head to catch some momentum to swing up into sitting. Keep your knees bent, and your back and your chin tucked in. Now, rock and roll while keeping your knees close to your chest and using your core muscles.

● **Breathe out** as you roll back and breathe in as you move up.

● **Practise up to 10 times,** synchronising your breath with your movement.

Do your best to ignore any farting noises and just keep rocking!

Flapping Fish Pose (Matsya Kridasana)

This pose is a very relaxed, restorative yoga exercise, which you can practise while lying on your bed. The gentle pressure on your belly can release gas, stimulating your abdominal peristalsis. Sometimes this exercise can feel easier on one side than the other.

● **Lie on your front** with your left upper arm underneath your right ear and interlace your right and left hand. Bend your left leg sideways, bringing your left knee close to your ribs while keeping your right leg straight. Try to rest your left elbow as close as possible to your left knee.

● **Close your eyes and relax** in this pose for a couple of minutes, before changing sides.

● **Occasionally yogis fall asleep** during this exercise. Don't worry if you do – it is fine and obviously what you need.

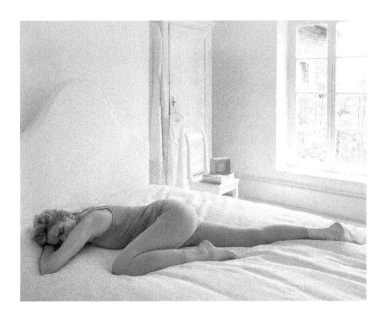

FURTHER TIPS

● **Fennel seeds** can help to reduce gas, bloating and stomach cramps. Chew half a teaspoon full of plain (not sugarcoated) seeds after each meal.[3]

● **Probiotics and prebiotics,** containing beneficial bacteria, can help with a bloated belly.[4]

● **Stop drinking through a straw** and hydrate the old-fashioned way – drinking directly from the glass. As you suck through the straw, you are inhaling air into your belly, creating the perfect storm for gassy conditions.

● **Smoking** is very similar to sucking through a straw. And electronic cigarettes are not any different – you will still be swallowing a good amount of air as you inhale.

● **Don't eat when you are nervous** or in a hurry because when you eat fast you swallow too much air.

● **Try massaging your abdomen** in a clockwise motion and that may help to get rid of trapped gas, reducing cramps and bloating (see Constipation chapter, p.63). First massage and then relax with a hot-water bottle on your tummy.

● **Ask your GP** about hyoscine butylbromide. I sometimes take these anti-spasmodic tablets when my belly is bloated because of IBS (irritable bowel syndrome).

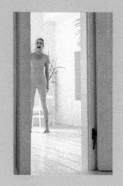

Getting old

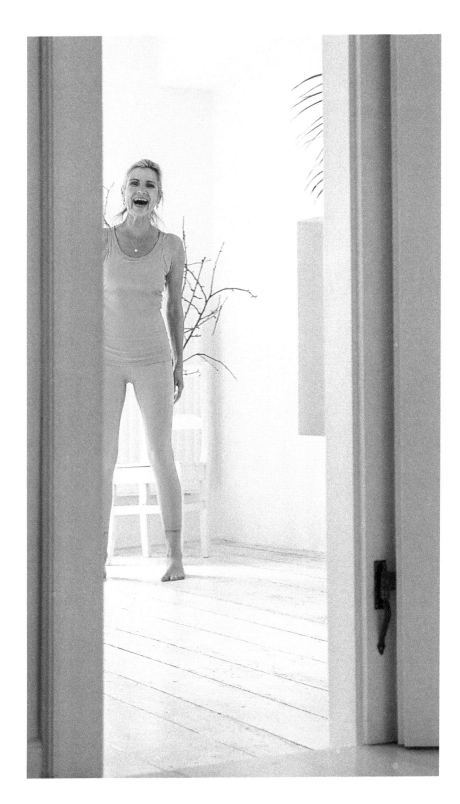

Getting old

"Old age ain't no place for sissies!" [1]

Bette Davis (Actress)

Getting old is an inevitable part of life that holds no alternative: you either get older or you die.[2]

While I appreciate this, occasionally I find this privilege of aging rather challenging. Every morning I can identify a new issue in my body: my belly feels bloated, my eyesight is getting worse, my brain cannot process and distinguish information as quickly, and concentrating has become a real task.

Nevertheless, despite all the aches, pains and concerns, I can find happiness in getting old. Helping me are the *Tibetan Rites*, a sequence of exercises I have been practising for the last 50 years. I truly believe that these rites are the reason why I still look and sometimes feel younger than I actually am. It is never too late to introduce these rituals into your life …

Known as the Tibetans, the ancient rites don't get nearly as much credit as they should. They are also referred to as the 'Fountains of Youth' or the 'Rites of Rejuvenation'.[3]

Studies have shown that practising specific yoga exercises can be a way to slow down the aging process and to maintain, or even improve, physical and mental wellbeing while getting older.[4] Research suggests that the flexibility of your spine can also help with the flexibility of your arteries. Therefore, a yoga practice such as the Tibetans, which is centred on suppleness of your spine, can keep your arteries in a more youthful state.[5] Simply devote up to 15 minutes of your precious time and practise the Tibetan Rites every morning.

Each rite is meant to be repeated 21 times, but start doing them just 3 times during the first week. Add 3 repetitions per rite in the following week. Continue adding 3 repetitions per rite each week until you are doing 21 rounds of each rite every day. However, when you don't feel like doing 21, feel free to stick to fewer repetitions.

Why 21 repetitions? In Tibetan culture, odd numbers are regarded as fortunate, and the number 21 seems to have some special spiritual significance. Furthermore, according to research, 21 grams is the physical weight of the soul. It is calculated by measuring the body weight of patients immediately before and after their deaths.[6]

All the exercises in this chapter are deceptively simple yet powerful, so build up slowly, listen to your body and modify as necessary. I have modified the original rites to protect more vulnerable body parts, such as the neck and lower back. You can further amend each ritual to suit your body and condition.

Caution: Please be aware that when you watch the Tibetan Rites online, people sometimes overstretch their necks, and copying this could cause more harm than good.

At the end of this chapter, I have included a meditation exercise, which also can unblock and speed up your *Chakras*, energy centres (see p.328).

EXERCISES

Spinning (first rite)

Remember when you were a kid, being unconditionally happy and spinning around just for fun? Well, that's exactly what you are going to do in this exercise. It can be a bit scary at first, but I promise you that you will quickly appreciate the positive impact of this practice on your brain, balance and movement.[7]

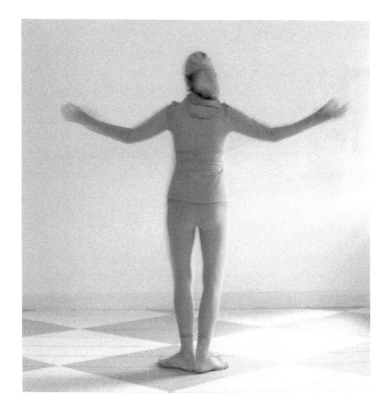

Caution: Do not practise this exercise if you suffer from vertigo, high blood pressure or any neurological disorders. Take extra care if you are doing this exercise when pregnant.

I always turn clockwise because turning anti-clockwise seems unnatural and makes me feel a bit sick. The idea behind clockwise spinning is that it can speed up your chakras, which can slow down with age.[8] Keep your eyes wide open throughout the spinning, letting your vision blur until you stop. Then immediately look at something right in front of you, for example your hands. If you spin for too long or go too fast, your brain can react with nausea and dizziness. This reaction is normal because your brain is protecting itself from too much input.

● **Stand with your feet parallel**, hip-width apart and extend your arms in line with your shoulders. Bend both your legs slightly, keeping your spine upright and your shoulders relaxed. Now, turn from left to right, spinning clockwise, gradually increasing the number of spins. Ideally start with 3 rotations, slowly building up to 21. You may feel a bit dizzy but you will eventually appreciate this feeling of freedom and happiness that kicks into your system while you spin around.

● **To finish,** instantly bring your hands into a prayer position right in front of your face, focusing your eyes until any dizziness you might experience disappears. Then, lie down and wait until your heartbeat returns to normal.

MODIFICATION (EASIER)
Stand in Mountain Pose (see p.78) with your arms relaxed and your feet hip-width apart. Lift your left heel and rotate your upper body to the right, breathing in, back to centre, breathing out. Repeat 3 times to the right, then to the left. Next, turn from side to side 3 times, breathing in through your nose, turning to the right, breathing out through your mouth, turning to the left. With time, increase up to 21 times. Always keep your eyes open. When finished, focus on your hands right in front of your face.

Leg Raises (second rite)

Leg raises can be tricky because people can try to compensate for the weakness of their core by overworking their lower back. Therefore, I suggest that you put a yoga block underneath your tailbone, your lower back, and lift just one leg at a time. Once your core muscles are stronger, you can raise and lower both legs. Always listen to your body and don't force anything.

● **Lie on your back with your legs bent** and your feet off the floor.

● **Straighten both legs, in line with your hips.** Press your lower back into the floor or block. Look at the ceiling and push down your shoulders. Breathe in. There is no need to lift your head.

● **As you exhale, slowly lower one leg,** pressing your lower back into the floor. Then breathe in, lift the leg again and exhale, lowering the other leg. Repeat 3 times, eventually working up to 21 times.

● **To finish,** hug both legs into your chest and gently roll from side to side.

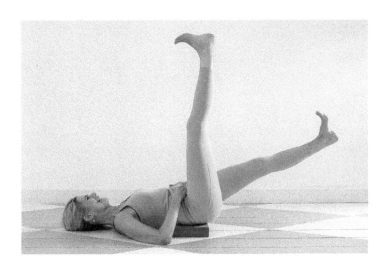

Kneeling Backbend (third rite)

A backbend can be stimulating and is often associated with the attitude of embracing life. Furthermore, gentle backbends can help to prevent back conditions, keeping the spine flexible. Place padding under your knees if they are sensitive.

Caution: Do not practise with severe back pain, knee problems or a hernia. Be careful when you have an overactive thyroid. Do not tilt your head if you have any neck problems.

● **Kneel upright** and curl your toes under. Tilt your pelvis slightly forwards and squeeze your bottom.

● **Inhale, lift your shoulders up,** back and down while moving into a gentle backward bend. Keep squeezing your buttocks as you lift your breastbone, arching your spine.

● **Breathe out ,** return to neutral and tuck in your chin. Relax your bottom.

● **Then, squeeze your bottom again,** roll your shoulders, breathe in through your nose and come into a backward bend. Breathe out through your mouth and return to neutral.

● **Repeat a couple of times** up to a maximum of 21 times.

● **Relax** in Child's Pose (see p.241).

MODIFICATION (HARDER)
Known as the Camel, this is a strong backbend. You can try it once you have done the above exercise 21 times. Make sure that you do not let go of your feet, especially when you enter and exit the pose. Only release your hands once you are sitting back on your heels, not before. This technique will prevent you from abruptly twisting your spine while exercising a backbend.

- **Sit on your heels,** toes curled under, with your spine straight, your hands on your heels and your thumbs on the inside your feet.

- **Lift your hips,** without letting go of your hands and push your pelvis forward, squeezing your glutes.

- **Lift your breastbone** and keep your head neutral or look up to the ceiling, neck permitting.

- **Hold the pose** for a couple of breaths, focusing on a deep in-breath.

- **Exit the pose** by sitting back down on your heels, without taking your hands off your feet.

- **To finish,** let go of your feet and stretch out on all fours.

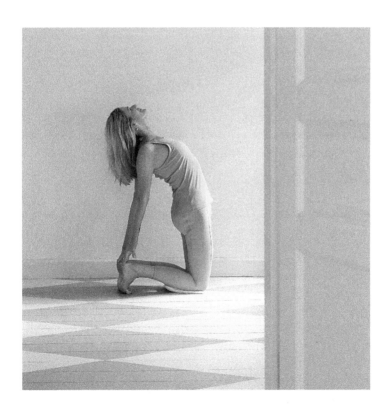

Reverse Tabletop (fourth rite)

This exercise is easier when using two yoga bricks or books placed next to your hips.

Caution: Do not practise if you suffer from recent or chronic injury to knees, hips, arms, back, shoulders or neck. Never drop your head lower than your shoulders.

● **Sit on the floor** with your legs extended and your feet hip-width apart.

● **Straighten your spine** and put your hands on the bricks next to your hips, fingers pointing forwards.

● **Inhale, bend your legs** and swing your hips forwards and up. By doing so, you come into a reverse tabletop position with your feet parallel, flat on the floor. Squeeze your bottom and keep your hips in line with your knees. Tuck in your chin.

● **Exhale, swing back** and return your buttocks in-between the two bricks, lifting your chin slightly.

● **Move between the 2 positions** as steadily and fluidly as possible and in harmony with your breaths.

● **Repeat 3 times,** eventually working up to 21 times.

● **To finish,** bend your legs, round your spine and relax your arms and shoulders.

ALTERNATIVE (EASIER)

This alternative is ideal for people with weak wrists and less upper body strength. Sit on the edge of a chair with your hands on armrests, lifting your bottom up and down, while keeping your spine straight and not bending forwards at any time. Inhale as you go up, exhale as you come down.

Child/Dog (fifth rite)

This true heart opener is slightly modified from the original Tibetan exercise, and gentler on your lower back. Most important: take your time and work with a long in- and out-breath. Take a normal in- and out-breath when you return to neutral.

● **Kneel and sit back** towards your heels as if in Child's Pose (see p.241).

● **Stretch out your arms,** with your hands on yoga bricks, and relax your forehead on the floor, with your chin tucked in. Don't worry if your bottom doesn't touch your heels.

● **Inhale and swing forwards** so your shoulders are above your wrists and your torso lengthens and opens into a back arch, looking forward. Your knees remain on the floor.

● **Exhale and return to the starting position**, while rounding your spine and releasing your hips back onto your heels. Breathe in and out, then take a deep breath in and start another round. Start with 3 times, working towards 21 repetitions.

● **Work very slowly,** as you straighten, round and arch your spine. When finished rest in Child's Pose for a few minutes, feeling the energy you have created, and allowing your breath to settle.

I believe the Tibetan Rites
are the reason why I still
look and sometimes feel
younger than I actually am.

Abdominal Lock (sixth rite)

The recommendation that this rite should only be practised when you feel an excess of sexual energy might explain why a lot of people practise just 5 Tibetan Rites.[9] The sixth one was probably designed to control the sexual desire within the Tibetan monk community …

I have included this exercise, not because I want you to have less sex, but to increase your inner fire and strengthen your pelvic floor and abdominal muscles to improve your sex life!

I never practise more than 3 repetitions. Perform this exercise early in the morning before breakfast.

Caution: Don't do this exercise if you are pregnant, or if you have high blood pressure or glaucoma. Be careful if you have reflux.

● **Stand with your feet hip-width apart and breathe in.** Now, while you powerfully breathe out through your mouth with pursed lips, bend your legs and place your hands on your inner thighs, with your elbows pointing outwards and your fingertips inwards.

● **Do not breathe in again but hold your breath.** Suck in your navel towards your spine, creating a vacuum. Tilt your pelvis slightly forwards, squeezing your butt, rounding your spine, and gazing down at your belly button, which is sucked in towards your spine.

● **Hold the lock for as long as you can hold your breath,** then release the muscle contraction *before* you take a deep breath in again, coming back up. If you try to breathe in before you release the abdominal muscles, you may start coughing. Try again twice before you lie down and relax.

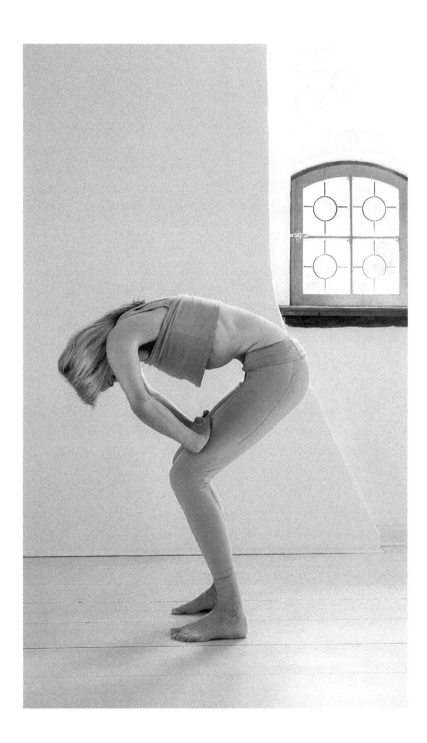

Chakra Meditation

There seems to be evidence that regular meditation can slow down the process of aging, at least at a cellular level.[10] I love a chakra meditation because it helps me to feel more balanced and focused. You can do this meditation, lying or sitting, maybe wrapped up in a shawl. Make this your time, with nobody interrupting you for the next 5-10 minutes. Ask a friend or your partner to guide you through this meditation or record it on your phone and play it back.

Your body is full of energy, *Prana*. This life force travels through thousands of channels, called *Nadis*. What the veins are for blood, the *Nadis* are for *Prana*. *Nadis* culminate and come together in *Chakras*, energy centres, which are all over your body (see p.328). In this meditation we are going to focus on the 7 main chakras along your spine, with the intention of making them spin faster again.

● **Lie down on your back** and start the journey at the base of your spine, which is the seat of your *Muladhara Chakra*, the Root Chakra. This is the region where *Kundalini*, your spiritual energy, is located.

● **I would like you to visualise this energy centre** in a velvety red colour. Imagine a red ball spinning at the base of your spine.

● **Move a bit further up** and see a vibrant orange ball spinning. Orange is the colour of the *Swadhisthana Chakra*, your Sacral Chakra. It is located just below your navel, and it is the seat of your emotions, sexual energy and creativity. Picture a spinning orange ball in your lower abdomen and back.

● **Now, imagine a beautiful golden sun**, spinning right at the centre of your body, supplying you with warmth and energy. This is your *Manipura Chakra*, the seat of your willpower, control and confidence, radiating its energy to all the chakras above and below your navel.

● **Move up to your chest** and visualise a striking emerald, green colour. The green leads you to your Heart Chakra, the *Anahata Chakra* - yogis sometimes call this the 'Sea of devotion and love'. Picture an emerald green ball spinning evenly in your chest and upper back.

● **Slowly, let go of the green colour and picture a light,** mid-blue, leading you to the *Vishuddha Chakra*, your throat and neck energy centre. This is the seat of communication and self-expression, affecting how you present yourself to others and how others perceive you.

● **From the light blue,** move up to see an indigo blue colour, leading you to the point between your eyebrows, the *Ajna Chakra*. This is the so-called 'Third Eye', seat of intuition and clarity of thought.

● **Envision a deep, blue-coloured ball,** spinning fast and evenly between your eyebrows and the back of your head.

● **Eventually,** the deep indigo-blue turns into a lush purple colour, leading you to the top of your head, the *Sahasrara Chakra*. Strictly speaking this is not a chakra, but your entrance to eternity.

● **Picture a purple-coloured ball** turning clockwise above your head.

● **Finally, see all the colours again:** the red, orange, yellow, green, blue and purple. Imagine a magnificent rainbow above your body with all its colours: the velvety red, the bright joyful orange, the strong sunflower yellow, the rich emerald green, the light mid-blue of the sky, the deep indigo blue and the purple.

- **Like the colours of the rainbow**, the 7 main chakras and their colours can exist in harmony, complementing each other.

- **The energy centres spinning evenly,** unblocked and freely, can help you in finding your equilibrium, the balance between getting older, living in the moment and looking forward to the future.

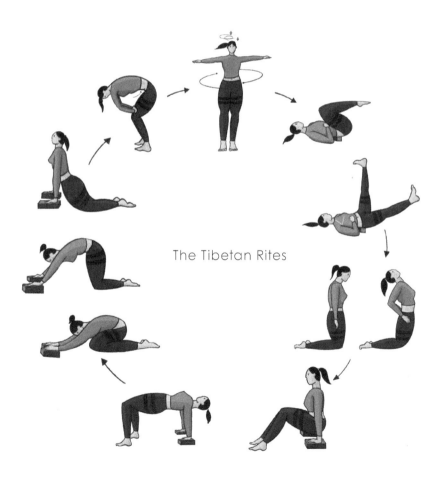

The Tibetan Rites

FURTHER TIPS

● **Try to enjoy sex.** Research reveals that sex can make us all look years younger and boosts our immune system and mood.[11]

● **Stay curious.** The moment you lose your curiosity and interest in your surroundings, you are officially old.

● **Walk tall.** Good posture is the best medicine to feel and look young.

● **Do not let anyone persuade you** that any aspect of ill health, from chronic pain to depression, is 'to be expected' in later life. It is not. Get any health concerns checked out and/or ask for a second opinion.

● **Drink lots of water,** even if you are not feeling thirsty. Water is essential for nearly every bodily function, from lubricating your joints to regulating body temperature and pumping blood to your muscles.

● **Use tinted moisturiser** to look healthier. Make-up and powder settle into wrinkles and can accentuate them, making you look older than you are.

● **Have a look** into the amino acid L-arginine. The anti-aging benefits look promising.[12]

● **Vitamin B12 and omega-3** fatty acids can improve or delay decline of your brain capacities. Vitamin B12 is important for cognitive functions in older people.[13]

● **The oldest** and healthiest people in the world live in Okinawa, Japan. They eat little saturated fat, salt or sugar.[14]

● **Enjoy a daily taste** of assorted cognitive tasks, such as Scrabble, Wordle or Sudoku. You may feel that you have more control over your cognitive abilities by working them.

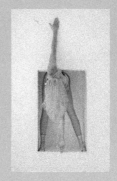

Hair loss

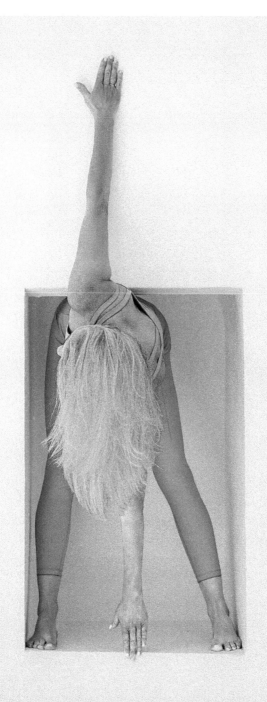

Hair loss

"A woman who cuts her hair is about to change her life." [1]

Coco Chanel (Fashion Designer)

The first time that I became fully aware of the importance of hair and the fear of losing it, was when I did a documentary for German television about dying. For most of the female cancer patients I interviewed, the loss of their hair seemed to be more traumatic than the probability of their deaths.[2] It was heartbreaking to see how hair loss upset these women to such an extent that they even considered abandoning lifesaving chemotherapy because of it.

Even though hair does not perform any vital function, its psychological importance is immense. Women who experience hair loss often talk of suffering embarrassment and low self-esteem, as well as feeling inferior and unfeminine.[3] Although men seem to cope better with hair loss – probably because it is more expected and accepted – its effects can still be incredibly upsetting.

In the UK, an estimated 8 million women suffer hair loss. An online poll of 1,700 women, conducted by the ITV show *Loose Women*, found that 94% claimed that hair loss was a worry for them.[4]

There are lots of possible reasons for hair loss. It is always good to consult a doctor to exclude any underlying illnesses, e.g., polycystic ovary syndrome, iron deficiency or thyroid problems. But hair loss is most likely down to genes or hormonal imbalances.

My hair was always thin and fine and one of the first things that popped into my head when I was pregnant with my first daughter was 'Please let her have more hair than I do.' And, indeed, she was born with a head full of black hair. Sadly, she managed to lose lots of it during her teenage years because of drastic bleaching and her hair is only just recovering from these treatments.

When you don't have much hair, even a short episode of hair loss can be upsetting. Once you have excluded fundamental causes and there seems to be no medical explanation for your hair loss, try to stay positive and patient. I know this can be a real challenge, but it is essential to stay calm because more stress can increase hair loss.[5]

What you can do is literally take matters into your own hands. *Balayam Yoga* is an ancient Indian practice. With *Balayam*, you vigorously rub your fingernails against each other. This sends a message to your brain, which in turn signals the adult stem cells present in your hair follicles to initiate the process of producing new hair follicles or to begin the rejuvenation of your damaged hair follicles.[6] There are no risks in trying this and no costs involved, so why not find out for yourself if nail rubbing works or not?

I also suggest doing some yoga inversions, upside down poses, for example the Downward-facing Dog, or a forward bend. There is no scientific proof that upside down poses help against hair loss but just like a head massage performed twice daily, you stimulate the blood flow to your scalp and that can help to initiate new hair growth.[7]

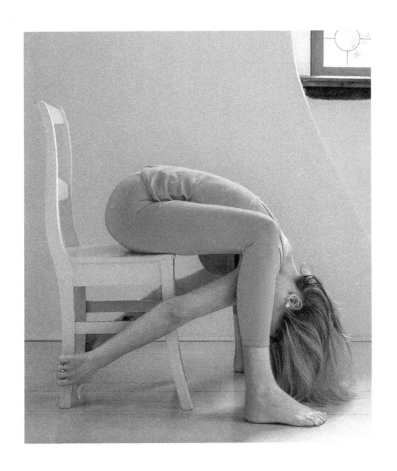

Even though hair does not perform any vital function, its psychological importance is immense.

EXERCISES

Nail Rubbing
(Balayam Yoga)

You can practise this simple exercise as often as you like - for example, when sitting at your desk or while watching TV. It is best to practise it twice daily for 10 minutes. Do not expect wonders, but hopefully after a couple of months you will be able to see a difference and new hair growing at your hairline.

Caution: Do not practise this technique when pregnant, if you have high blood pressure or if your nails are infected.

● **Sit comfortably.** Place your hands at chest level, tucking your elbows into your ribcage. Then, curl your fingers inwards so that they point towards your palms.

● **Bring your hands together** so that the nails of all the fingers, not your thumbs, are in contact with each other. Rub your nails against each other vigorously, so that the nerves in your nail bed can get a good amount of friction.

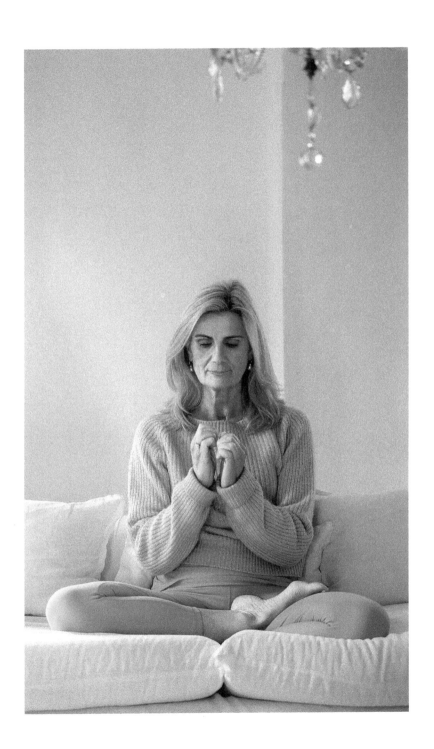

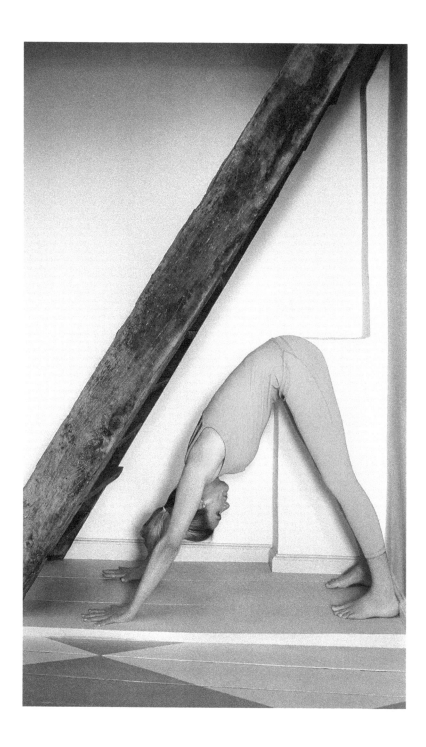

Downward-facing Dog
(Adho Mukha Svanasana)

This pose can help to stimulate more blood circulation in your scalp, which then hopefully strengthens your hair follicles and, over time, promotes hair growth.

Caution: Do not practise inversions if you suffer from high blood pressure, vertigo, glaucoma or any recent or chronic injuries to your neck and shoulders.

● **Position yourself on all fours** and spread your fingers apart, bringing your head slightly further forwards. Curl your toes under and lift your knees a couple of inches off the floor, while keeping your legs bent.

● **Now, focus on lifting your hips upwards** and drawing your chest towards your thighs. It is not essential to straighten your legs. Keep your legs slightly bent if you need to and try to bring your chest closer towards your thighs. Relax your head.

● **Breathe in through your nostrils** and breathe out through your mouth, with a soft sighing 'Ha' sound. Repeat up to 10 times.

● **To finish, gently drop your knees** onto the floor and relax in Child's Pose (see p.241) before repeating the exercise again.

Rabbit Pose (Meditation)

I like to practise this posture on an acupressure mat with hundreds of little spikes, but I realise this may not appeal to everyone.[8] The Rabbit Pose can, of course, be performed on a normal yoga mat, or directly on the floor, just as well.

● **Kneel and place your forehead** on the floor or mat. Position your hands either side of your head and lower your bottom onto your heels. Relax, then lift your hips while keeping your head on the floor or mat. Now, roll from your forehead onto the crown of your head. If you are using the acupressure mat it may cause a bit of pain, but you will get used to it.

● **Once you are on the crown of your head,** your arms should be creating a right angle with your elbows pointing behind you and your thighs should be almost vertical to the floor. Then, drop your bottom back down. Lift your hips and roll forwards onto the crown of your head again. Keep moving up and down, without taking your head off the floor or mat. Inhale as you bring your bottom back and exhale as you move forwards. The more you roll forwards and backwards, the better. Start with 5-10 repetitions, aiming to increase to 21.

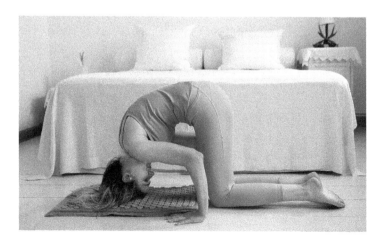

FURTHER TIPS

- **Whenever I notice** that I start losing more hair than normal, I take minoxidil, the only scalp treatment that helps me to reduce hair loss.[9] It is available without prescription and can be used by men and women. However, it is likely that you will lose your hair again once you stop using minoxidil.

- **To improve** both hair thickness and hair growth, rosemary oil seems to be an excellent choice, thanks to its ability to improve cellular generation.[10]

- **Whenever I wash my hair,** I like to finish with ice-cold water! It is refreshing, can decrease hair loss and makes my hair shine.[11]

- **Some people** see a lot of hair-growth potential in Korean Red Ginseng, which can be taken as tea or capsules.[12] Another benefit of ginseng is that it can work as an aphrodisiac.

- **The hair on your head** might get thinner with age, but your facial hair can get more visible. Get a magnifying mirror and get rid of any unwanted hair around the chin and upper lip.

- **Sleep on a soft cushion** or pillowcase made of mulberry silk. This is supposed to be good for skin and hair and feels divine.

- **Invest in a real hair piece** or clip-in hair extensions, but avoid weave-in extensions. The constant pulling can cause strands of hair to break or to fall out.

- **If you dye your hair,** always do a patch test first. Ensure the dye doesn't contain PPD (paraphenylenediamine), an allergen that has been linked to hair loss.[13]

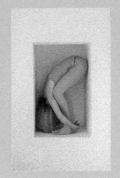

Hangovers

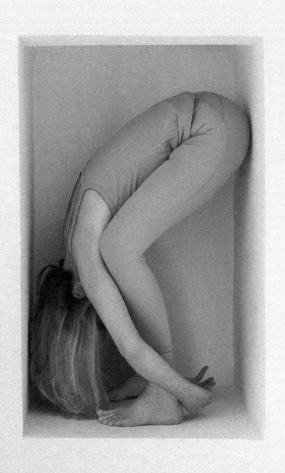

Hangovers

"I have taken more out of alcohol than
alcohol has taken out of me." [1]

Winston Churchill (Politician)

am the daughter of an alcoholic and, from an early age,
I witnessed how my father's alcohol abuse affected my
parents' marriage and ruined our family life and business.
One of the most upsetting experiences for me was when my
father tried to stop drinking and the withdrawal led to delirium
tremens, a psychotic condition involving perceptual
distortions, tremors and disorientation. My mother was
absent, so at just 10 years old, I had to deal with my
hallucinating and rambling dad on my own. That was scary.
There is no getting away from it: drinking to excess is bad for
your health and your relationships. And the fear connected to
these memories will accompany me for the rest of my life.

Decades later and, despite my experiences, surprisingly
I enjoy drinking. However, I am a bit of a lightweight and 3
glasses of red wine is my limit. Even then, the following day is
awful with headaches, nausea and brain fog - simply a wasted
day, with me moaning and feeling very sorry for myself.
Thankfully, this does not happen too often because, as we get
older, we show a tendency to experience fewer hangovers.[2]

However, it appears that the symptoms of the hangover itself can worsen with age, possibly because our metabolism slows down and the liver takes longer to eliminate toxins.

As well as affecting us personally, hangovers can impact the whole economy. In the UK, health problems in connection with alcohol cost the NHS up to £2 billion a year and, according to new research, hangovers cost the economy up to £1.4 billion a year.[3]

There is no real cure for hangovers, unless you decide to stay off booze completely, which I know is not feasible for lots of people. Therefore, I want to share some tips and yoga exercises that can help you to get over a hangover faster, reducing the negative side effects of too much alcohol consumption from the night before.

The first rule is to stay hydrated during your evening out, always alternating a glass of alcohol with a glass of water. This simple trick can help to minimise major future hangover symptoms. Make sure that you drink still water, as sparkling can make you drunk even faster.[4] Before you go to bed drink at least 1 pint of water and another when you wake up early in the morning. This will probably be at around 4am because this is the time when your liver tries to get rid of the alcohol in your body. Make sure to replenish with even more water during the day, adding some electrolytes (e.g., sport drinks) and eat something salty or a banana to replace the salt and potassium you lost from drinking too much alcohol.

Although you might not be in the mood, it is worth doing some gentle stretching the morning after, either in the form of sex or yoga exercises. Alcohol by the way, can increase your sexual desire and arousal, but only up to a certain point. After more than 2 drinks the alcohol in your blood will have a more negative effect on your sex drive.[5] William Shakespeare was spot on when he wrote: 'It provokes the desire but takes away the performance'.[6]

So, what kind of yoga exercises can you do after waking up with a hangover? Start with single nostril breathing - the Sun-piercing Breath, *Surya Bhedana,* can purify the frontal part of your alcohol-infused brain and is more efficient than a cup of strong espresso.

Furthermore, the great Master of Yoga, B.K.S. Iyengar, suggested that twisting yoga exercises help to detox your body. Iyengar called this the 'squeeze and soak' action - squeezing the inner organs like a wet sponge, so that the liver and the kidneys expel old blood and allow fresh, richly oxygenated blood to take its place. As much as I like this idea of fresh, rejuvenated inner organs after a boozy night out, sadly there is no real scientific proof for Iyengar's theory. Yet, I always felt that gentle yoga exercises, including twists, helped to ease my hangover symptoms.

Don't feel tempted to sweat out your hangover with a hot yoga or *Bikram Yoga* session, because heat can cause further dehydration. Also, avoid doing inversions (upside down positions) because usually there will still be too much acidity in your body, and it may cause you to feel sick.

Instead, be kind to yourself and practise *Ahimsa* (non-violence), one of yoga's ethical principles. Accept the self-inflicted weakness, try not to feel guilty and make allowances for yourself for the rest of the day.

EXERCISES

OPTIONAL PROPS
Tissues to blow your nose, 2 yoga blocks or a bolster, blanket

Sun-piercing Breath (Surya Bhedana)

This breathing technique can stimulate your sympathetic nervous system, heat your body and help to remove toxins. Only your right nostril is used for inhaling, stimulating the left side of your brain. If you need more energy, speed up. Practise for no longer than a minute in the beginning.

Caution: Do not practise if you have high blood pressure or any kind of heart disease. If you feel dizzy, slow down.

● **First, blow your nose** with a tissue.

● **Sit with your spine as straight as possible.** Relax your face and shoulders.

● **In a moment, you will be inhaling** solely through your right nostril and exhaling through your left nostril.

● **Place the ring finger of your right hand** against the side of your left nostril to block it. Inhale through your right nostril. Then, close the right nostril with your right thumb and exhale through the open left nostril. Close your left nostril again to breathe in through your right nostril. Continue inhaling right and exhaling left for a minute.

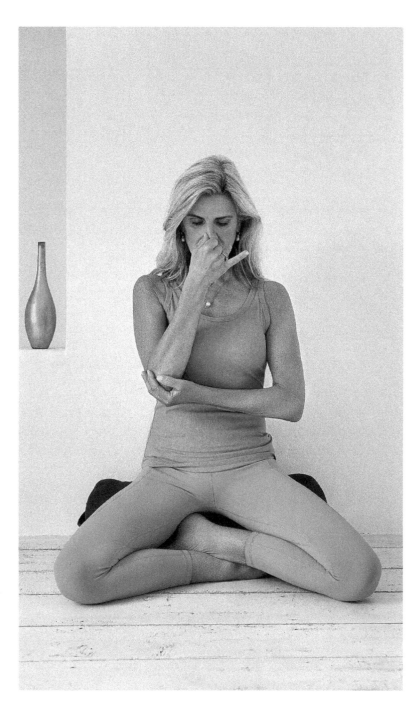

Child's Pose (Balasana)

This is a posture to rest and relax, so make it as comfortable as possible and hold the pose for as long as you like. There is no need to rush. Let go of any toxic thoughts – there have been enough toxins in your system. You may want to put a few drops of essential oil on a tissue – ginger, peppermint, and lavender may help to ease your hangover symptoms.[7]

- **Kneel on the floor.** Bring your big toes together and sit on your heels. Then, either separate your knees or keep them together. Whatever feels better.

- **Lean forwards so that your forehead touches the floor.** If your head cannot reach the floor, rest it on 2 yoga blocks. If your bottom cannot reach your heels, place a folded blanket behind your knees.

- **Decide whether to extend your arms** out in front of you or keep them close to your body.

- **Focus on deep breathing,** while gently elongating your spine. Slowly roll your forehead from side to side, inhaling the uplifting and refreshing oil, if you are using it, without getting the oil too close to your eyes.

- **If you feel sick,** lift your head and focus on a long in-breath and out-breath. If you are feeling okay, you might want to move your arms further forwards, stretching out even more.

- **Come into a seated position** with both your legs extended out in front of you. Lift your arms, give yourself a further stretch and get ready for a gentle twist (see opposite page).

Seated Twist (Ardha Matsyendrasana)

To get the most out of twists, always start the rotation from your navel, and not from your head or chin.

● **Extend your legs** out in front of you. Now, bend your left leg to cross it over your right leg.

● **Bring your left hand behind you** and lengthen your spine. Bring your right hand around your left knee and start to rotate from the navel to the left. Look forward at your big toe as you gently rotate first from your navel, then ribcage and shoulders and, finally, your head and chin. Move slowly, using your hand on your knee to gently increase the twist.

● **Inhale as you elongate and exhale as you rotate.** Hold the twist for 3 breaths, then gently release and move first your navel, ribs and then your head back to centre. Repeat the twist on the same side before you do 2 twists to the right.

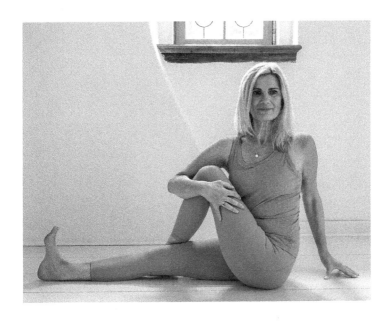

Moon-piercing Breath
(Chandra Bhedana Pranayama)

In this breathing technique only the left nostril is used for inhaling. This breath can quiet the right, more emotional side of your brain.

● **First, blow your nose** with a tissue.

● **Come into a seated position** of your choice with your spine as straight as possible. Relax your face and shoulders.

● **Now, block your right nostril** with your right thumb and inhale very slowly through your left. Then close the left nostril with your right ring or index finger and exhale through the right nostril. Close the right nostril and breathe in through your left nostril. Continue in a slow manner, inhaling left, exhaling right, inhaling left, exhaling right for 1 minute.

● **Rest for a moment before you get up** and take a shower. Then simply relax on the sofa and drink some warm ginger tea.

Accept the self-inflicted hangover, try not to feel guilty and make allowances for yourself for the rest of the day.

FURTHER TIPS

● **Get your timing right.** Winston Churchill, who drank 6 glasses of champagne or wine daily along with whiskey or brandy never seemed to be suffering a hangover, simply because he drank over a period of 15 hours, and his body had enough time to absorb the alcohol.[8] Now, I don't want to encourage you to start drinking in the morning, but I want you to take your time and not to drink too much too quickly.

● **Try to 'meditate' with alcohol.** Get a glass of wine, look at its colour, sniff its aroma and then very slowly take a sip. Taste the delicate bouquet, swirl the wine in the glass for a 'second nose', noting more flavours, and then swallow. It might take half an hour for you to finish your glass this way, but you are less likely to have a hangover the next morning because by drinking more mindfully, you will drink less.

● **Use a tongue scraper** to get rid of the fluffy tongue feeling and stale breath that accompanies a hangover.[9]

● **Never drink on an empty stomach.** Make sure that your meal includes carbs that can 'soak up' the booze.

● **Catch up on Vitamin B12 and B1.** Also, artichoke is supposed to be helpful in supporting your liver function.[10] Another off-the-shelf supplement that may be a hangover cure is NAC (N-acetylcysteine), usually given to asthmatics. It seems to help and improve hangover symptoms especially in women.[11]

● **If you are concerned** about someone's drinking, or indeed your own, contact the free and confidential alcohol helpline Drinkline. In the UK Tel: 0300 123 1110 weekdays 9am–8pm, weekends 11am–4pm, or speak to your GP.

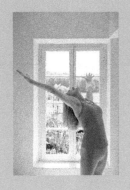

Happiness

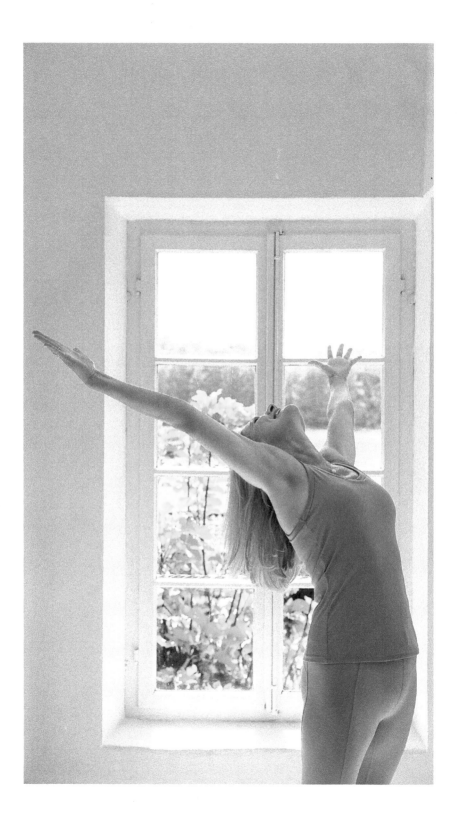

Happiness

"Be happy. It really annoys negative people." [1]

Ricky Gervais (Comedian)

What makes me happy? Little things like sniffing a baby's head, wearing a new dress, a child smiling, the scent of freshly cut grass, flowers in my garden, oven-warm bread with salty butter, a dip in the ice-cold sea, laughing with friends, and falling asleep in my husband's arms whilst watching a romantic comedy.

Relationships and positive human interactions are a great source of happiness. Sadly, throughout the Covid-19 pandemic, when I began writing this book, there were not many opportunities to enjoy each other's company and this unusual isolation evidently affected all of us: the average happiness level in Britain deteriorated to its lowest level, and anxiety increased to the highest levels on record. [2]

Throughout my life, I've experienced episodes of sadness, often triggered by something somebody said or did, unfairness or the fear of not being loved or good enough. Most times, I manage to crawl out of my hole and regain equilibrium - my inner balance. I accept that there are happy and less cheerful times. I probably wouldn't appreciate one without the other.

I can't magically create contentment, but there are happiness-inducing exercises I do, and that I can share with you: my 'happiness routine'. Yoga exercises such as spinning (see p.129)

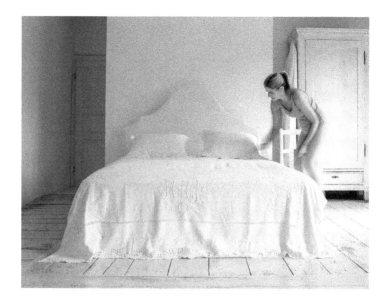

and loud sighing out-breaths are part of this routine and so are basic things like making my bed in the morning.[3] The theory behind this is to accomplish at least one thing every day. Starting my day by completing the simple task of making my bed gives me a feeling of *Santosha*, contentment.

It helps that I get up early. It has been established that being a morning person is associated with better mental health and more happiness. Whereas people who prefer the evening hours are more prone to depression.[4] Even though it is sometimes hard, I try to ditch being a night owl and instead engage with my inner morning-lark.

The next recommendation may sound unbearable, but it works for me: start the day with a cold shower. The exposure to cold water can activate the sympathetic nervous system and increase your level of feel-good hormones, endorphins. Also, due to the high density of cold receptors in our skin, a cold shower can send an overwhelming number of electrical impulses to your brain, which could result in an anti-depressive effect.[5]

If the cold water doesn't appeal to you, then try to clap your hands, ideally while listening to a catchy tune. This works for both kids and adults. Hand-clapping songs can improve your motor and cognitive skills. Once you start clapping, you will feel more positive and alert.[6]

Finally, the most important tool: smile! Smile as soon as you open your eyes in the morning - even if you wake up thinking: shit, another awful day. A big fat fake smile can trick your brain into believing that you are happy, even when you are not. A fake smile can kickstart actual feelings of happiness, setting off mood-boosting chemicals in your brain. So, you can quite literally fake it till you make it.[7]

If a fake smile triggers feel-good hormones, think of how much more effective a truly deep belly laugh can be. Laughing on cue might not come naturally to you, but it is easy to learn. A marvellous way to increase your happiness level is to practise something called *Hasya Yoga*, laughter yoga, either alone or in a group.[8] If you are interested, there are more than 10,000 laughter yoga clubs worldwide and about 25 in the UK.

Now, with a big smile on your face, I invite you to explore the other yoga exercises in this chapter. Some are a bit more challenging and may move you out of your comfort zone but sometimes we need to dare ourselves to feel happy.

And, remember, whatever you do, try to do it consciously. Any attentive activity can increase your happiness levels. Dancing, singing, making love - all these actions can stimulate the production of serotonin, the happiness messenger, when done mindfully.[9, 10]

EXERCISES

Shoulder Balance

No risk, no fun? If you are reasonably fit, take a risk and try something that feels a bit different. After all, what will happen if you lose your balance? Not much, you will simply roll onto your backside and start again.

Caution: Do not attempt this exercise if you are pregnant or suffering from osteoporosis, or have shoulder or neck problems.

● **Position yourself on all fours.** Take off any glasses.

● **Lift your right arm** and rotate your upper body to the right side, looking at your hand, your palm pointing away from you. Now, swing your arm under your chest, through the gap between your left shoulder and left knee, something we call 'threading the needle'.

● **Relax on your right shoulder** with the side of your head on the floor or on a block. Your right arm extends out to the left. Extend your left arm forwards beyond your head and relax in this upper spine rotation.

● **Next, bring your left hand back in front of your face,** you will need your fingers to balance in a moment. Lift your left leg, without opening your hips. Explore how far you can lift your leg without losing your balance. And if you do, just laugh it off as you roll onto your bum, and then start again!

● **If you like the balance, keep the left leg lifted** and lift your left arm as well, balancing on your right shoulder and knee. To hold the balance, try to keep your lifted arm in line with your shoulder. Hold the pose for a couple of breaths, then release your arm and leg. Repeat on the other side.

If you lose your balance, don't worry – just laugh it off as you roll onto your bum, and then start again!

Tree Pose (Vrksasana) against a wall

This pose is less 'tricky' than the Shoulder Balance but an equally happiness-inducing exercise. It is not just about mastering balancing on one leg, but about feeling grounded and being able to expand and grow at the same time.

● **Stand with your feet hip-width apart** against a wall in the Mountain Pose, *Tadasana* (see p.78), with just your buttocks touching the wall.

● **Stand tall with your arms at your sides** and as you inhale, bring your weight onto your left leg. Lift your right leg and place the sole of your foot onto your inner left thigh, calf or ankle. Avoid the knee joint. Shift the weight from the outside of your standing foot more to the inside, lifting your kneecaps and engaging your inner thigh muscles.

● **Bring your hands together in *Namaste*.** Press your left big toe into the ground and imagine the roots of your tree being embedded deep down in the earth.

● **Slowly raise your arms overhead,** extending every finger upwards. Touch the wall behind you with the tip of your thumbs and move your bottom away from the wall. If you like, bring your thumbs and index fingers together, into *Chin Mudra*.

● **Keep looking straight ahead** and find a *Drishti*, a steady gazing point, that can help you to focus and maintain your balance. Lifting your upper body and your arms can be a transformative moment in which you feel happy, free and light.

● **Try to hold the posture** for at least 1 minute, with a big smile on your face.

● **To finish, release your hands** back into *Namaste*, release your leg and then repeat the exercise on the other side.

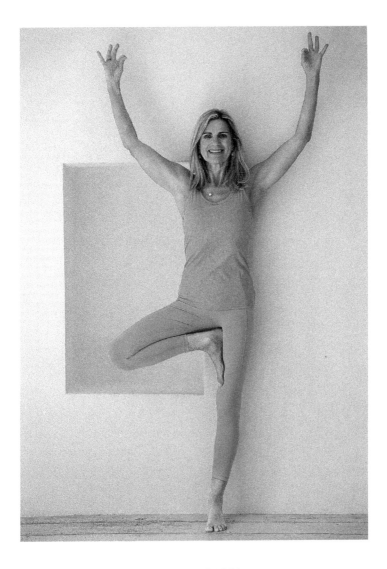

MODIFICATION (WITH A PARTNER)

Partner up with someone - preferably someone of a similar height - to do the Tree Pose. Stand side-by-side, close enough to each other that your hips are touching. Now, bring one arm around each other's waist and bend your outer leg out to the side. Hold the pose. Performing this double Tree Pose together is fun, instantly creating happiness and laughter.

Laughter Yoga (Hasya Yoga)

I remember how awkward I felt at my first Laughter Yoga session. But once I dared to let go and not judge myself, I thoroughly enjoyed the experience. I hope you will like it too.

● **Stand and clap your hands together** as if applauding yourself. There doesn't have to be a specific rhythm – simply feel the warmth and energy that you are creating whilst clapping.

● **Move your hands over to one side clapping twice,** then to the other side, again clapping twice. Continue going from side-to-side, clapping for 30 seconds.

● **Now, produce a sound as you are clapping:** say 'Ho Ho' to one side and 'Ha Ha' to the other side. Clap and sing along for a couple of minutes.

● **To finish, lift both your arms into the air,** breathe in deeply and breathe out with a 'Ha' sound, releasing your arms down again.

● **When you release your arms again, start laughing.** Produce a lovely fake laugh, ideally right from your centre. The hope is that eventually this fake laugh will turn into a beautiful natural belly laugh.

MODIFICATION (WITH A PARTNER)

First, do the sequence above with your partner. Then, lie down and place your head onto their belly. Start laughing together, while your head rests on your partner's belly. This will increase feelings of happiness once you allow your minds and bodies to harmonise.

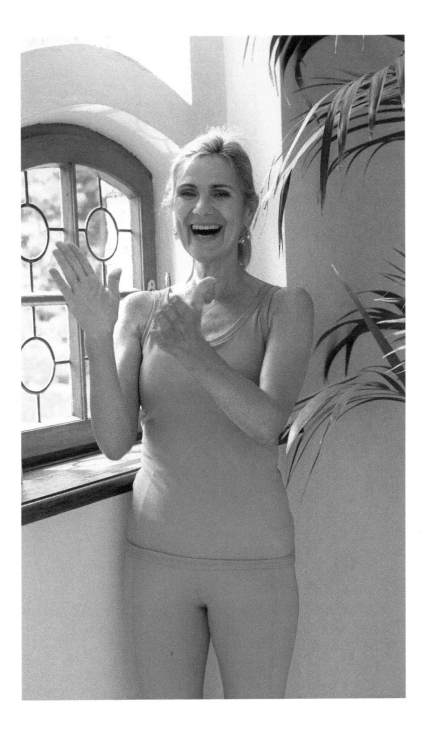

Chocolate Meditation

Meditating with extra dark chocolate (approximately 80% cocoa content) can be powerful and fun. The reason is that dark chocolate contains phenylethylamine, a neuromodulator that can lift your mood and decrease cortisol levels, the stress hormone that often leads to anxiety and mood swings.[11, 12] If chocolate is not your thing, replace it with something else, perhaps raisins or gummy bears, or a glass of red wine.

Either ask a partner to read out the meditation or record yourself saying it and play it back.

● **Sit comfortably,** on the floor or on a chair with your spine straight, and a piece of dark chocolate to hand.

● **Hold the chocolate** and look at its colour, shape and texture. Don't eat it yet!

● **Then, close your eyes and smell the chocolate** – its strong fragrance. Notice how your mouth starts watering. Swallow, open your mouth, and place the chocolate onto the tip of your tongue. Close your lips and move the chocolate very slowly from side to side. Simply enjoy this sensuous delight of tasting and eating chocolate, feeling no guilt – just pleasure.

● **Sit quietly.** Your head is relaxed, your spine straight. Touch your tongue on the inside of your upper teeth and then rest your tongue against your inner lower teeth.

● **You may have swallowed the chocolate already** or still have a little bit left in your mouth.

● **Once the chocolate has gone completely,** notice the strong after-taste.

● **Now, inhale deeply,** and exhale with a soft 'Ha' sound. Let go of the chocolate taste with each out-breath, but hold onto this feeling of contentment for a bit longer.

Gayatri Mantra

Some people find peace and happiness in chanting, while others might not experience the same effect. I personally like to feel the vibration when chanting this mantra.

Om bhur bhuvah svah

tat savitur varenyam

bhargo devasya dhimahi

dhiyo yo nah prachodayat.

The eternal, earth, air, heaven

That glory, that resplendence of the sun

May we contemplate the brilliance of that light

May the sun inspire our minds.[13]

This mantra can be practised by anybody, anywhere, anytime to bring a feeling of contentment.

Happiness-inducing Songs

Listening to music and singing can make you feel happy. Create your own list of happiness-inducing songs. Here are some of my favourites, which you might want to try out:

- *Good Morning Blues* (Tom Jones/Jools Holland)
- *La Donna è Mobile* (Luciano Pavarotti and friends)
- *Uptown Girl* (Billy Joel)
- *Bella Ciao* (Manu Pilas)
- *The Power Is Here Now* (Alexia Chellun)
- *Let's Dance* (David Bowie)
- *That's Life* (Frank Sinatra)
- *What A Wonderful World* (Louis Armstrong)
- *September* (Earth, Wind & Fire)
- *Downtown* (Dusty Springfield)

FURTHER TIPS

● **Don't resist change** – it is important. People who are fearful of change are rarely happy. It doesn't have to be a massive change, just enough to keep your life interesting and stimulating.

● **Try to help and care for others.** Helping others will make you feel happier, unless you always expect something in return.

● **Poke the universe** and take risks.

● **Spin around clockwise.** Remember when you were a kid, feeling happy and spinning around just for fun? You can still do this as an adult (see p.129), and it can evoke strong feelings of happiness. No one manages your happiness, except you.

● **Have a regular digital detox.** Ignoring social media for a couple of hours, or more, can lift your spirits.

● **Fill your home** with the uplifting scent of fresh lemons. Buy some good quality lemon or lemongrass oil, put it in a diffuser and the pleasantness of the scent can make you feel happy.[14]

● **Enjoy sex.** Sex with more awareness can increase your happiness, whereas unwanted sex can lower your happiness.[15] It is about quality, not quantity.

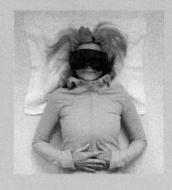

Insomnia

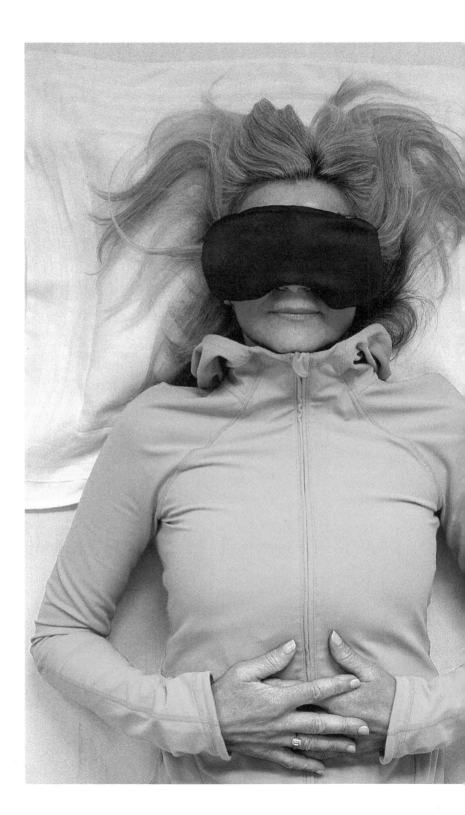

Insomnia

"A ruffled mind makes a restless pillow." [1]

Charlotte Brontë (Novelist)

When I was little, I never wanted to sleep. I was afraid of the dark and the possibility of not waking up again. As a student I preferred to study at night and when I worked as a radio journalist, I was happy to do night shifts.

I was content with an average of 4-5 hours sleep per night, until I had kids. Then, my sleeping pattern had to change. I couldn't keep up with the lack of sleep. Over the years, I have managed to transform more into a morning person, sleeping approximately 6-7 hours per night. I can fall asleep more easily, but I often wake up at around 3am and find myself tossing and turning, looking for a position that can help me to go back to sleep. To make matters worse, I start to resent my husband, who is snoring gleefully, oblivious of my struggles.

Sleep deficiency is exasperating and can make you feel and act like a zombie. Satisfactory rest and sleep play a fundamental role in the effective functioning of your body, and a persistent lack of it can create a significant risk not just to your physical, but also to your mental health.

Compared with good sleepers, insomniacs suffer way more chronic health problems, including heart and kidney disease, high blood pressure, diabetes, obesity and depression. Therefore, it comes as no surprise that studies have found that chronic sleep deprivation is linked to a greater overall risk of death![2]

And it bothers a lot of us. In the UK, insomnia is estimated to affect a third of people at some point in their lives. It tends to be more common among women and more likely to occur as people get older.[3]

The first step in addressing sleeplessness is to allow an expert to rule out any underlying medical causes. However, it often turns out that insomnia is simply the result of an over-active mind within an over-stimulated nervous system. Yoga's sister science *Ayurveda* believes that a hyperactive mind is the cause for most sleeping problems, often affecting people with a *Vata*-dominated constitution (see p.330).

If you are governed by *Vata*, you tend to be all over the place: quick, intelligent and often with a nervous constitution. You would certainly benefit from more steadiness and stability in your life, including a regular yoga practice, which should then positively affect your sleeping habits.

Furthermore, everybody deprived of sleep should invest in some personal 'sleep hygiene', a term used to describe healthy habits that can influence your ability to fall and remain asleep. Some examples of good sleep hygiene are getting up every morning around the same time, including weekends, regardless of how poor your night's sleep has been. Avoiding daytime naps after 3pm and opting for a brisk walk instead. Eating regular, ideally warm, comforting food and avoiding eating late into the evening. Stopping work 2 hours before you want to fall asleep. Banning smartphones (unless used for sleeping apps), action movies, or anything over-stimulating from your bedroom – with one exception: sex.

Studies have shown that orgasms with a partner or through self-stimulation were associated with the perception of better sleep quality.[4] Sexual activities before bedtime can make you fall asleep easier, whereas yoga can assist with the continuity of your sleep.

Yoga can help you to relax your body, reducing common causes of insomnia, such as stress and anxiety. Therefore, it has a positive effect on sleep quality and the severity of insomnia.[5]

My favourite exercise when waking up at around 3am is the Rabbit Pose (see p.152). I roll forwards and backwards on the crown of my head on an acupressure mat around 50 times, focusing on my breath. After this, I am able to go back to bed and fall asleep.

The ideal yoga exercise in the evening is the Supported Shoulder Stand against the wall. Another gentle approach to being upside down is legs up against a wall. Any inversion can stimulate your pineal gland; this 'magic' pea-sized gland in your brain produces and secretes melatonin, a hormone that can help to regulate your sleep cycle.[6]

Another efficient tool not to be missed is *Yoga Nidra*, a deep relaxation. Your mind remains conscious, but your entire body relaxes as if you were asleep. *Yoga Nidra* can help with anxiety, depression and the management of chronic insomnia.[7] It doesn't replace the missing hours of sleep, but with the help of *Yoga Nidra* you can feel as refreshed as if you have had sufficient sleep, and it can prepare your body and mind for a good night's sleep.

EXERCISES

Standing Forward Bend (Uttanasana)

The great Master of Yoga, B.K.S. Iyengar, once said that after practising *Uttanasana* 'one feels calm and cool, the eyes start to glow, and the mind feels at peace'. This is exactly how I would like you to feel after practising this gentle forward bend.

Caution: Do not practise any inversion if you have unmedicated high blood pressure, severe acid reflux or glaucoma. If you suffer from lower-back pain, be extra careful and make sure that you keep your knees slightly bent.

● **Stand upright**, with your bottom against a wall.

● **Your feet should be parallel,** more than hip-width apart, and approximately 1ft away from the wall. Keep your legs slightly bent as you curl down vertebra by vertebra from your hips, lower back, middle part of your spine, finally releasing your neck and head. Forget about being able to 'touch your toes'; this is not what this posture is about. Instead, relax your upper body, arms, head and neck, and feel blood rushing into your head. Stay in the forward bend for a moment with your eyes closed – simply relax. Letting go, try to accept sleeplessness rather than obsessing over it.

● **To move back up,** vertebra by vertebra, first press your feet firmly into the ground and engage your leg muscles, then slowly curl your way up, taking your time. Repeat the exercise twice more.

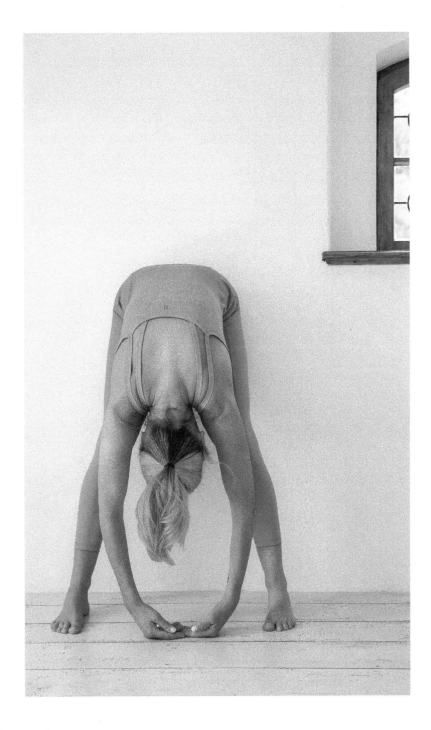

Shoulder Stand
(Sarvangasana) in 3 stages against the wall

The Shoulder Stand is sometimes called the Mother or Queen of all postures because of its soothing and nurturing nature (see Stress chapter, p.283). Using a wall will allow you to enter and exit this pose safely, without demanding too much of your core strength. There should be no cushion underneath your head.

Caution: Do not practise this exercise if you have severe neck problems, osteoporosis, untreated high blood pressure, glaucoma or severe acid reflux.

● **Sit down on the floor,** with your right hip against a wall and your legs bent.

● **Now, swing your legs round,** roll onto your back and bring your legs up against the wall.

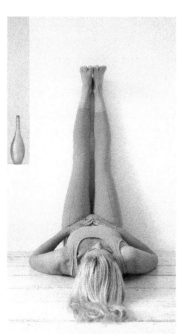
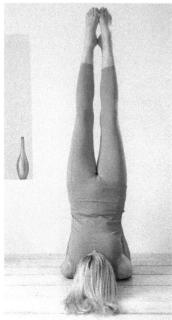

- **Shuffle your bottom** as close to the wall as possible.

- **This may be as far as you want to go today.** Relax and enjoy or move into the Half Shoulder Stand.

- **Bend your legs,** pushing the soles of your feet against the wall.

- **Lift your hips off the floor,** creating a right angle with your legs and upper body.

- **Now, support the back of your pelvis** with both your hands and keep the elbows in line with your body. Press both your feet firmly against the wall and feel the impact on your pelvis moving forward. Squeeze your buttocks but relax your facial muscles, your jaw and neck. Again, this may be as far as you want to go. If you like, stay in this stage of the pose for a couple of minutes, simply listening to your soft snoring sound of *Ujjayi* Breath (see p.84).

- **If you want to come into the full Shoulder Stand Pose,** release first one leg away from the wall, then your other leg, and eventually both legs. Try to keep your legs vertical, in line with your hips. Hold the posture for a couple of breaths, then bend your legs again and bring your feet back against the wall, slowly walking down the wall.

- **To finish, lie back on the floor,** separate and relax your knees to the side, keep the soles of your feet together and your chin slightly up.

Yogic Sleep (Yoga Nidra)

Regularly practising *Yoga Nidra* can promote a more restful and rejuvenating sleep.

● **Find a comfortable position** with your head supported on a yoga brick or cushion and your eyes closed. Rest your hands either beside you or on your lower belly. Take a moment to make any last adjustments so that you feel comfortable and at ease.

● **Silently recite a *Sankalpa*,** a short, positive statement. For example: 'I am okay and look forward to a good night's sleep'. Allow the *Sankalpa* to arise from your desire to nurture yourself and state it 3 times silently.

● **Take a deep breath in through your nose** and a sighing breath out through your mouth. Repeat this a couple of times.

● **Then, begin the journey through your body.** Firstly, bring awareness to the top of your head. Feel a sense of relaxation, as if a gentle wave of calm is washing over your scalp.

● **Now, shift your attention to your forehead.** Notice any sensations you may feel there. Relax the point between your eyebrows and allow your forehead to smoothen.

● **Notice the weight of your eyelids.** Let them be heavy and at ease. Your eyes are now deeply relaxed.

● **Shift your attention to your jaw.** Release any clenching or tightness. Relax the tip of your tongue against the inside of your lower teeth. Soften your lips.

● **Slowly bring your attention to your neck and throat.** Feel any tension leaving your neck and throat.

● **Sense any burden or heaviness** in your shoulders. Let go and feel your shoulders sinking into the floor.

- **Notice the rise and fall of your chest.** With each breath, your chest expands and contracts peacefully.

- **Move your awareness to your arms,** down your fingertips. Feel a pleasant heaviness in your arms as they rest.

- **Guide your attention to your belly and lower back.** Let go of any tightness and tension stored in this area. Feel a sense of calm and ease spreading through your core.

- **Shift your awareness to your hips and pelvis,** letting go of any toughness with your out-breath. Allow your lower body to feel light and comfortable.

- **Bring your attention to your thighs, knees and calves.** Relax your legs and feet, your ankles and toes.

- **Simply rest in a peaceful state**, soon allowing yourself to transition into sleep. Repeat your *Sankalpa*, your positive statement again. Echo the same statement you made at the beginning and silently repeat it 3 times, nurturing your deeply planted wish for sleep and healing.

- **Go to bed.** Put lavender, clove or geranium oil on your pillow or wrist and focus on your breath. Inhale through your nose for 4 and exhale through your nose for 8. Continue for as long as you like, though you may find yourself nodding off …

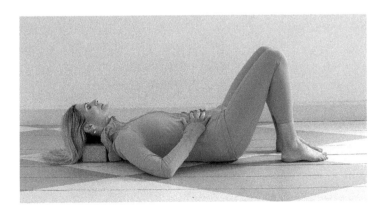

FURTHER TIPS

● **Try taking an anti-histamine** instead of sleeping pills. There is a study that shows that antihistamines, containing chlorpheniramine, can act like an anti-depressant and help you to sleep better.[8]

● **Look into GABA**, a neurotransmitter supporting your sleeping rhythm. Contact your GP if in doubt, or if you are pregnant or you have any underlying thyroid problems.[9]

● **Enjoy alcohol** but not as a sleeping aid. Alcohol can help you fall asleep, but overall it is more disruptive to the quality of your sleep, particularly in the second half of the night.[10]

● **Take magnesium,** melatonin and a vitamin B complex in the evening. Studies indicate that 3 months of a magnesium-melatonin-vitamin B complex supplementation has a beneficial effect on the treatment of insomnia regardless of cause.[11]

● **Take a warm bath** before you go to bed, with 12 drops of rose oil, 12 drops of geranium oil and 12 drops of lavender oil.[12]

● **When you wake up in the middle of the night:** get out of bed, have a cup of camomile tea or a decaffeinated tea with a bit of cinnamon and oat milk. Nutmeg, cardamom pods, cinnamon and honey all have sedative qualities, helping you to relax.

- **Sleep separately from a snoring partner.** Of course, we love them but sometimes they can ruin our sleep. Better move them into another room (if available) or at least let go of the large duvet and cuddle up in single duvets with the aim of falling asleep before the snorer.

- **Remember that your bedroom** should be cool and dark and meant for sleeping and sex only. Unless you are listening to one of the many sleep-inducing meditations. Choose the one with a voice you like that makes you feel comfortable, safe and sleepy.

Invest in some personal sleep hygiene – healthy habits that can influence your ability to fall and remain asleep.

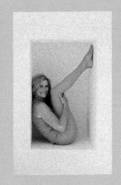

Menopause

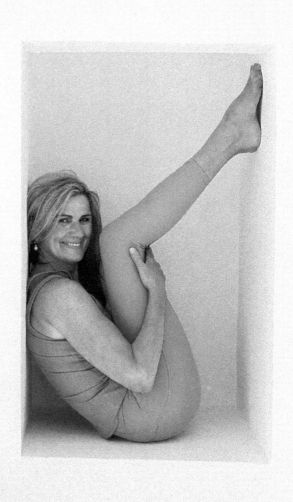

Menopause

"Menopause can be the best time of your life ... where you don't care what people think about you." [1]

Julie Graham (Actress)

A lack of libido, vaginal dryness, bladder infections, hot flushes, mood swings, fatigue, insomnia, osteoporosis, a fat belly and itching skin: these are just some of the more than 30 symptoms that women can develop during menopause. For some, menopause is a smooth transition, while for others it can pose a decade of great discomfort with several of the above signs being so severe that women even consider giving up on significant aspects of their lives, such as their relationships and jobs.

Women are often surprised not only by the irregularity of their periods, but the irregularity of their emotions. Several studies have found an increased incidence of depression and anxiety in women during the menopausal transition, due to the often drastic fluctuation of their oestrogen levels. [2]

Menopause can be divided into 3 stages: perimenopause, menopause and post-menopause. One-third of the entire UK female population, around 13 million women, are currently perimenopausal or menopausal, meaning that they are either about to transition or in the middle of it. Menopausal women are the fastest growing demographic in the workforce. The Equality Act 2010 states that although the menopause is not an illness or disability, the effects can be disabling, meaning that employers who fail to properly support women could be found to be discriminatory.[3]

At the age of 45, I suffered 3 miscarriages within a year. The first 2 times I had to go home to bleed out the little embryo, which was cruel. The third time the baby stopped growing at around week 15 and I needed an emergency scrape and antibiotic infusions. Soon after this traumatic year and my last moments of fertility, my body drifted into menopause. And as if to confirm it officially, I received a letter from the NHS stating that the cause of all my miscarriages was age and no further investigations were worthwhile. Ouch, that hurt.

Hormone replacement therapy (HRT) is probably the most effective tool against most of the unpleasant menopausal symptoms. I was prescribed it because of the thinning of my bladder, making me prone to infections.

Taking HRT turned out to be the right decision for different reasons, mainly because, unknown to me at the time, I already had osteoporosis. As well as being a fertility hormone, oestrogen strengthens your bones and supports your heart and brain function. There is a small possibility that HRT can increase the risk of breast, ovarian and womb cancer, but I felt that the advantages of taking HRT outweighed this.[4] However, it is a personal decision, so talk to your GP about all options.

Now, in my mid-60s and barely using the hormone patches, I have noticed more physical and mental changes: my monthly cycle has finally stopped, my mood swings are slightly more aggressive, my body temperature seems to vary from freezing cold to boiling hot, and while my hair is falling out, new hair is growing in places where it shouldn't. Thankfully, because I continue having an enjoyable physical relationship with my partner, I can bask in oxytocin, the love hormone, despite my low oestrogen and progesterone levels.[5]

It certainly helps to have a husband who is open to discussing the menopause, accepts the biological changes taking place, and who is not inclined to go for a younger, more fertile model. If you do not want or do not have a partner, try to befriend other like-minded people, sharing your physical, psychological and social experiences. Community, *Sangha*, can be a great source of healing.[6] There are numerous online platforms for menopausal women (see p.215); it can be comforting and informative to read what others describe and to contribute your own experiences.

Rather annoyingly, men do not go through menopause because their hormone levels decline slowly, if at all, and it doesn't involve a complete shutdown of their reproductive organs. With women, ovulation ends and hormone production plummets during a relatively short period of time, whereas men can still produce sperm into their 80s and beyond. However, sexual complications, such as lack of libido and erectile dysfunction, may arise as a result of lowered testosterone levels.[7]

So, now that talking about the menopause seems more acceptable, what can we do in order to feel and look better during these challenging years? Studies reveal that yoga can reduce some of the symptoms, improving your overall quality of life. Also, a regular yoga practice, for example 30 minutes every day over a couple of months, can naturally increase oestrogen levels.[8, 9] Though yoga cannot replace the loss of oestrogen, it certainly has its place in managing most of the symptoms caused by the decline of the hormone. The breathing, meditation and physical movements of yoga can

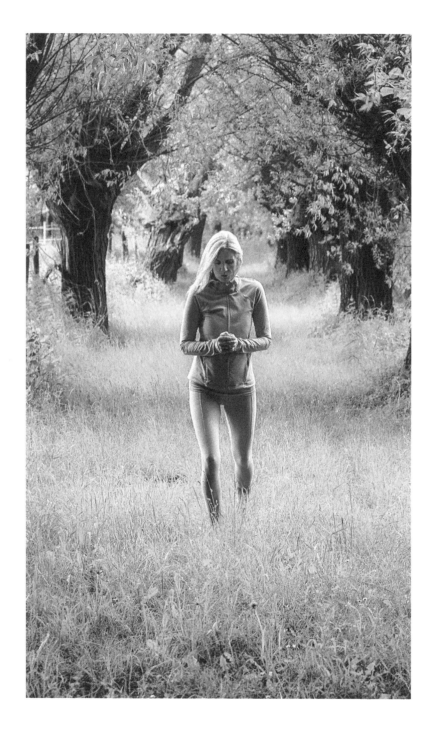

affect all parts of your body simultaneously. This is important because during menopause you can often feel several symptoms together.

The exercises I have picked for you particularly target mood swings, slow metabolism, hot flushes and a foggy brain. See specific chapters for exercises that target other symptoms, such as anger, fat belly, insomnia and lack of libido.

The first exercise in this chapter is part of *Pawanmuktasana* III, a group of yoga movements that can improve your energy, the functioning of your endocrines, and tone your pelvic organs and muscles.[10] In combination with first a slow breath, then gradually progressing to a more rapid breathing technique, this can be a beneficial way to deal with mood swings. Another great exercise is the *Kirtan Kriya*. Scientists are researching this *Kriya* to determine how it improves cognitive function and memory. Whether it is due to the breathing, visualisation, repetition of the mantra, or your finger movements, this exercise can clear a foggy brain.[11]

A regular yoga practice, for example 30 minutes every day over a couple of months, can naturally increase oestrogen levels.

EXERCISES

Stirring the Pot or Churning the Mill Pose (Chakki Chalanasana)

Practise this exercise in combination with the energising *Bhastrika* Breath (see p.320), which can stimulate your metabolism and digestive system.

Caution: Be aware that inhaling and exhaling rapidly can cause nausea and dizziness, but you can regulate these possible side effects by slowing down the speed of your breathing. Don't opt for *Bhastrika* if you suffer from high blood pressure, ulcers, hernia, epilepsy, asthma or heart disease. Don't stir the pot at all if you suffer from severe back pain. If you need to be careful of your back, practise the exercise while sitting on the edge of a chair.

● **Sit on a block or a book** with your legs approximately 2.5ft apart, keeping your spine straight. Interlock your fingers into *Kali Mudra*, a hand gesture that is believed to give you more energy to deal with difficulties and transformations. Your fingers are tightly linked, with your index fingers pointing away from you; your left thumb is crossed over your right, representing female power.

● **Now, imagine that there is a big pot of soup** or porridge in front of you, in-between your legs, and you are holding a massive spoon to 'stir the pot', using large circular movements. Keep your arms straight, at shoulder height and parallel to the floor – your index fingers should always be in line with the tip of your nose. Bend forwards from your hips and move to the right so that your hands pass above your toes. Then lean back keeping your arms up, rotating first over to the left and then to the right side, before leaning back again.

● **Continue making large circular movements** over both your feet. Point your feet as you move forwards and flex your feet as you move back. Try to move from your hips and not from the middle part of your back. Inhale through your nose while leaning back and exhale through your nose while moving forwards. Do not speed up; rather slow down, stirring the pot with awareness and in harmony with your breath.

● **If you cannot quite reach over your feet,** do not worry. Just make sure that you still hinge forwards from your hips and avoid rounding your spine.

● **Practise 5 rounds** clockwise and anti-clockwise, increasing up to 10 rounds.

● **Release your arms and relax your shoulders.** Roll them up, back and down a couple of times before you repeat the exercise. Alternatively, opt for a faster, more energetic round – this can lift your mood because you forcefully breathe in and out through your nose, *Bhastrika*, which can cause excitation followed by calmness.[12]

● **For the more dynamic round,** keep your legs just 1ft apart and your feet flexed. Extend your arms and quickly rotate from your hips, while keeping your upper body straight. Breathe in and out rather forcefully through both nostrils.

● **Practise up to 20 rounds** clockwise and anti-clockwise.

● **To finish,** lift your arms, interlace your hands and turn your palms up towards the ceiling. Hold your breath for a moment. Then, release your arms followed by a sighing out-breath.

Wide-legged Standing Forward Bend (Prasarita Padottanasana)

This calming exercise can provide all the benefits of a head stand, but is easier to accomplish. Practise this forward bend with 2 yoga bricks if you have tight hamstrings.

Caution: Do not practise this exercise if you have serious lower-back problems, glaucoma or high blood pressure.

● **Start in the Mountain Pose** (see p.78). Place your hands on your hips and silently jump your legs 3-4ft apart.

● **Engage your inner thigh muscles.** To do so, imagine that you are sitting on a horse using just the grip of your inner thighs. Make sure that your toes are pointing forwards and that the weight is on your big toes and on the outside of your heels.

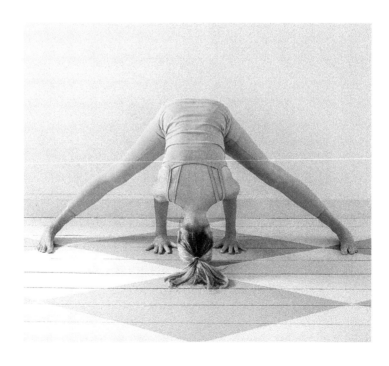

- **Now, bend your legs slightly** and hinge forwards from your hips, maintaining the length of your spine from the crown of your head to your tailbone. If you feel any discomfort in your lower back, stop and perform the easier modification with a chair (see below).

- **Then, fold further forwards,** placing your fingertips on the floor. You can pigeon-toe your feet further apart because the wider the stance, the easier it is for you to bend forwards.

- **Try to bring your hands in line with your feet.** Your fingers are pointing forwards and your elbows behind you. Relax your head down towards the floor. If you are using bricks, place the crown of your head onto a brick. If you cannot get your head near the floor, simply relax in the standing forward bend and focus on elongating your exhalation to your inhalation.

- **To exit the pose,** move your hands forwards, underneath your shoulders, bend your legs and pigeon-toe your feet back together. Relax your arms, keep your legs bent and slowly roll back up, vertebra by vertebra, and without your hands touching your legs.

MODIFICATION (WITH A CHAIR)
Place a chair in front of you. Positioning your hands at the front of the chair, bend your arms with your elbows pointing behind you and place the crown of your head (not your forehead) onto the chair. Relax in this pose without collapsing in your shoulders. With your head supported, the posture can feel very calming. Try to stay in the pose for a couple of minutes.

The Cooling and Hissing Breath
(Sitali and Sitkari)

The Cooling Breath can help to manage your night sweats and hot flushes. If you are unable to curl your tongue, you can practise the Hissing Breath, *Sitkari,* instead.

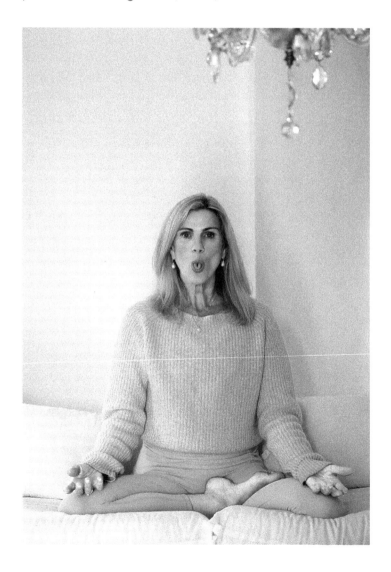

Cooling Breath (Sitali)

Sit comfortably, either on a chair or on the floor, with your spine straight, your shoulders relaxed and your chin parallel to the ground. Stick out your tongue and curl it lengthwise. Then, suck in the air through your curled tongue while slowly lengthening your neck. Close your mouth and breathe out through your nose while maintaining a long neck and a lifted breastbone. Repeat up to 10 times. When you are finished, instantly enjoy the calming coolness around your neck, throat and chest.

Hissing Breath (Sitkari)

Sit comfortably, either on a chair or on the floor, with your spine straight, your shoulders relaxed and your chin parallel to the ground. Smile widely with your teeth bared and touching. Breathe in through the sides of your mouth, then close your mouth and slowly breathe out through your nose. Repeat 10 times and then enjoy the calming coolness around your neck, throat and chest.

Cleansing Meditation
(Kirtan Kriya)

Try this thousands-of-years-old yoga practice to maintain your focus and possibly improve and protect your memory. You chant SA TA NA MA, changing your finger movements as you do so. Don't judge your chanting – the quality of your voice is not the point of this exercise!

Start practising each round for 1 minute without any pauses, then 2 minutes and, with time, increase up to 3 minutes, so that the whole exercise can last 9 minutes. Practise every day for 3–4 months and then evaluate the impact on your brain and memory.

- **Sit comfortably,** either on the floor or on the edge of a chair. Keep your spine upright and bring your arms out to the side at shoulder height to create cactus arms.

- **On SA,** press your thumbs against your index fingers.

- **On TA,** press your middle fingers against your thumbs.

- **On NA,** press your ring fingers against your thumbs.

- **On MA,** press your little fingers against your thumbs.

- **Continue the chanting and finger movements** throughout the exercise (use enough pressure so that your fingers blanch slightly) and your mind cannot help but stay focused.

- **Practise the first round for 1 minute.** Then, without a pause, lower your arms down and bring your elbows against your ribcage for the second round, when you move from loud singing to whispering SA TA NA MA.

- **Eventually, after another minute, start the third round,** repeating the chant internally in silence, while resting your hands in your lap, still pressing each finger against your thumbs.

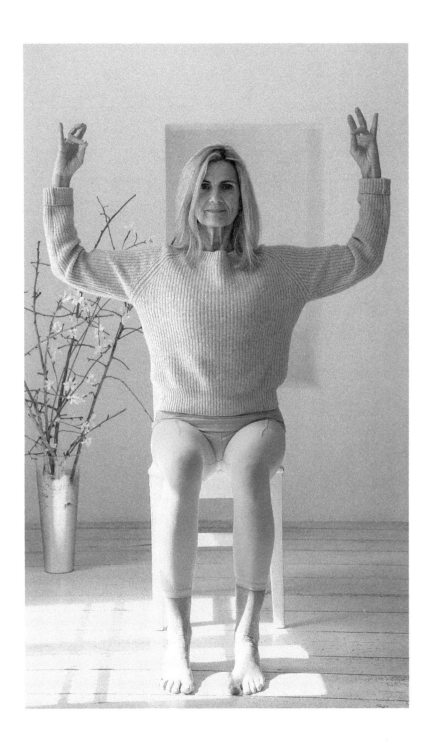

● **Now, take a deep breath in,** reaching your arms overhead. Exhale, draw your hands to your chest in *Namaste*. Repeat the SA TA NA MA mantra, which means 'truth is my identity', twice more.

● **To finish, consider using an essential oil,** including orange, cinnamon, cedarwood, sage or marjoram. These blends remind me of the transition time from summer to autumn. Rub the oil into your palms and wrists, but avoid direct contact with your face. Take a few deep breaths and relax.

MODIFICATIONS
If you have shoulder problems, practise the whole *Kriya* with your arms relaxed, your hands resting in your lap and your palms facing upwards.

If you like more of a challenge, finish the SA TA NA MA exercise and then practise the other way around, starting with your little finger and thumb and chanting in reverse order: MA, NA, TA, SA. By changing things up in this way, your brain cannot help but focus and improve!

Scientists are researching the *Kirtan Kriya* to determine how it can improve cognitive function and memory.

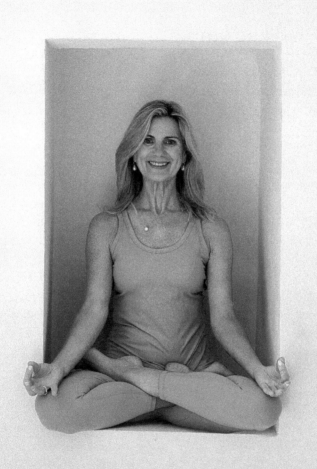

FURTHER TIPS

- **Accept menopausal changes.** Hot flushes last longer and are more intense when you try to resist them.

- *Ayurveda* **views hot flushes as a** *Pitta* **problem,** meaning there is too much fire in your body. To diminish *Pitta*, avoid consuming spicy food, hot drinks and alcohol (see Reflux chapter, p.253).

- **Spoil yourself with food you like,** boost essential fats and eat more phytoestrogens such as tofu, soy milk and miso. Studies have associated phytoestrogen intake with a slight increase in oestradiol in post-menopausal women.[13]

- **Look into reflexology.** There are indicators that regular reflexology can decrease anxiety, hot flushes and night sweats in menopausal women.[14]

- **Do you need to calm your nerves,** and minimise cramps and restless legs? Take a complete magnesium complex daily.[15] Also, enjoy tonic water with quinine, without or occasionally with gin. A low dose of quinine can treat nocturnal leg cramps.

- **To help to improve your cognitive health** and memory, look into taking a choline tablet daily.[16]

- **Clench your fists** every day to improve your memory. Unilateral hand clenching can increase the neuronal activity in the frontal lobe of your brain.[17]

- **Itching and dry skin?** Use soothing and cooling aqueous cream, also known as sorbolene.

● **Trouble sleeping?**
Discover the advantages of separate bedrooms. It also can work wonders for your sex life. A snoring or blissfully sleeping partner can be annoying, making your own symptoms feel worse. Therefore, if you have got the space, move into your own room (former kid's room?) and bed. Visiting each other for a cuddle can help to reinvent and stimulate your relationship.

● **If you are prone to getting bladder infections easily,** use a condom during sex because this can help to prevent cystitis. Furthermore, drink lots of water before and after intercourse.

● **Follow Dr Naomi Potter @dr_naomipotter.** A GP for 10 years, Dr Potter is now a specialist menopause doctor, approved by the British Menopause Society. From an empathetic female doctor's perspective, she frankly informs about menopause and recommends how to manage symptoms, creating a rather wonderful supportive community.

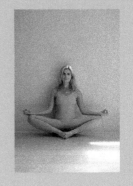

Osteoporosis

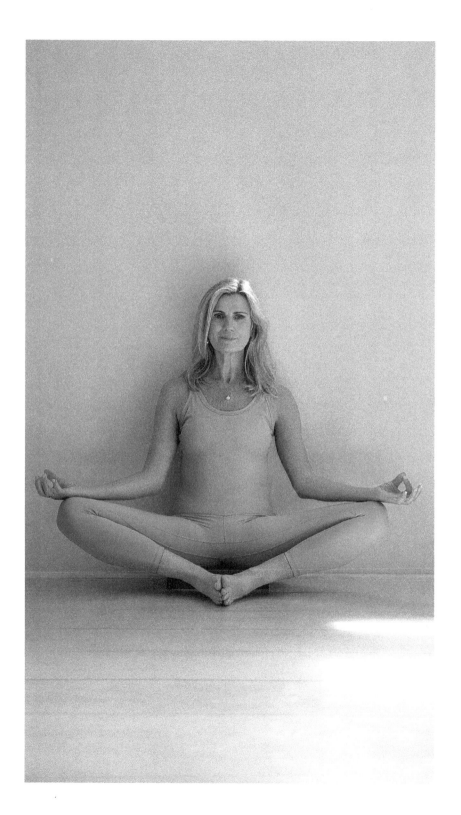

Osteoporosis

"Osteoporosis is one of the most urgent
societal challenges to living well in later life." [1]

Queen Camilla (Wife of King Charles III)

My beautiful, slender and stylish grandmother had a hunchback, a significant rounding of her upper spine, which made her look old and vulnerable, even though she was only in her late 50s. At the time, we didn't know that she had severe osteoporosis, the so-called 'silent disease'. It didn't cause her any discomfort until she experienced her first fracture, and then it all happened rather quickly. Several fractures and a weak heart eventually led to my granny's premature death.

If osteoporosis runs in your family, ask your GP to refer you for a bone density test. The earlier you know that you have got osteoporosis, or osteopenia (not yet osteoporosis), the sooner you can take preventative measures against it getting worse.

Loss of bone density is a big global health problem. In the UK alone, there are 3 million people diagnosed with osteoporosis and an estimated over 500,000 fragility fractures each year – that is roughly 1 every minute.[2]

Your bones are thickest and strongest in your early adult life, with bone mass being lost gradually from around the age of 35. This happens to everyone, but some people lose their bone density faster than others.

Various factors can contribute towards osteoporosis; the condition is more common in women than in men, with an early menopause increasing the risk. Certain illnesses such as rheumatoid arthritis, thyroid problems and conditions resulting in prolonged immobilisation can also increase the risk. Walking can regenerate your bones and a study found that consistently practising yoga can increase bone density even further. Also, yoga improves your balance and flexibility, which can prevent falls and fractures.[3]

So why, despite intense walking and a lifelong yoga practice, did I get osteoporosis in my legs, hips, back and neck? It is because of my genetic predisposition plus medication – reflux tablets – that I was advised to take for more than 30 years. This medicine, unknown to me at the time, prevented my body from absorbing essential vitamins and minerals. Long-term PPI (proton pump inhibitors) therapy, particularly at high doses, is associated with an increased risk of osteoporosis and fractures.[4]

However, without my life-long yoga practice it could have been much worse. Because of yoga, plus the recent extra intake of calcium and annual alendronic acid injections (see p.229), I actually managed to improve my condition.

There is not a one-size-suits-all solution when recommending yoga poses for someone with osteoporosis. Depending on how severe and where your osteoporosis is located, you may need to avoid doing sit-ups and crunches, and poses that require spinal flexion (rounded-back poses). If in doubt, talk to your yoga teacher before you start your practice. As a general guideline, it is best to avoid strong compressive or other forces on your neck, such as in head and shoulder stands. Instead, modify and practise yoga postures with the focus on lengthening your neutral spine.

Keep it simple and use light hand and/or ankle weights if you wish. Studies show that regular resistance training can help to prevent bone density loss and may even help to build new bone.[5]

In this chapter, I have also included *Kinhin*, a meditation technique that you might like to explore. It gets you moving but at the same time helps you to slow down, increase your balance and discover the beauty of moving forwards with more awareness. Staying active is important for bone health and osteoporosis, whatever your age or wellness and whether you have had broken bones in the past or not.

Consistently practising yoga can increase your bone density, as well as improve your balance and flexibility, which can prevent falls and fractures.

EXERCISES

Bridge Pose
(Dwi Pada Pitham) variations with weights

Because of osteoporosis, I suggest that you keep your spine as straight as possible as you lift and lower your back. You can practise this exercise with or without weights.

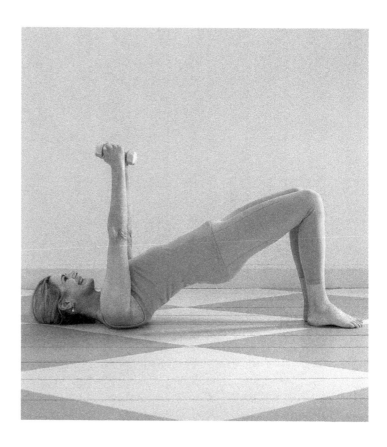

● **Lie on your back and bend your legs.** Keep your feet and knees parallel to each other, hip-width apart. Your arms are out to the side, shoulder height, a weight in each hand. Breathe in through your nose, lengthening your spine.

● **On your out-breath, lift your hips and chest** and come up into a bridge. At the same time lift your straight arms so the weights come together above your head. Breathe in and hold the posture, while squeezing your glutes and pushing your knees away from you. Make sure that your feet are parallel to each other, pressing firmly into the ground. Breathe out, release both arms and lower your back to the floor. Repeat 5 times.

● **Now, bring your extended arms with the weights over your head** behind you onto the floor. Your spine is flat on the ground and your legs are bent. Breathe in and lengthen your arms and spine. Breathe out, lift your arms and spine off the floor. Bring your arms forwards, towards your lifted hips, slightly above the floor.

● **Move your neck further away from your shoulders** and keep the back of your head (no cushion) in line with your lifted spine. Squeeze your glutes and push your knees away from you. Breathe in and move your arms back over your head, without touching the floor, releasing your flat spine back onto the ground. Repeat 5 more times. Practise slowly, focusing on long in- and out-breaths.

● **To finish,** hug your knees into your chest and roll from side to side, massaging your back into the floor.

Locust Pose (Shalabhasana)

This exercise can strengthen your back muscles, buttocks and legs. You can practise the pose with or without weights. Use a folded blanket under your hips for more comfort.

Caution: Avoid this pose if you have severe back problems.

● **Lie face down with your arms bent** and your elbows tucked into your ribcage. Tuck your chin under, lengthening your neck. This is your neutral position.

● **Now, breathe in**, press your pubic bone into the floor before you lift your head, chest and hands simultaneously. Keep gazing downwards, the back of your head in line with your spine.

● **Hold the pose for a couple of breaths,** while lifting your kneecaps, squeezing your glutes and lengthening your spine. The goal is to create a strong and long line from the crown of your head to your pointed toes, without lifting your legs. Breathe out and go back into the neutral position. Repeat at least 5 more times.

● **Alternatively, perform the lift holding weights,** with your arms extended and alongside your body.

● **To finish,** make a 'cushion' with your hands. Place your forehead on the 'cushion' and wiggle your hips a bit from side to side. Relax.

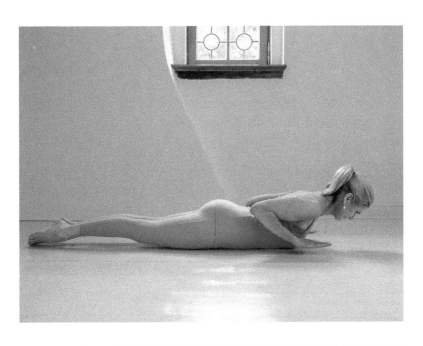

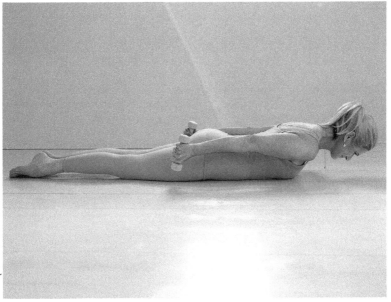

Mindful Walking Meditation
(Kinhin)

Make sure that you have enough space to walk in a fairly good size circle or oval. You can do this exercise in a group and turn clockwise in a circle 2m apart or practise it on your own. Ideally, do this walking meditation early in the morning barefooted in the garden or park.

In the traditional *Kinhin*, walking meditation, practitioners clasp their hands in *Shashu*, a grasp where the left hand is in a fist with the right hand covering it. *Shashu* represents focus and concentration. Alternatively, you can simply relax your arms.

- **Stand straight** with your feet at least hip-width apart. The gap between your legs will give you stability and balance.

- **Visualise yourself switching from a fast pace** to slow motion as you start walking, keeping your legs and feet hip-width apart throughout.

- **Move one leg forwards and land on your heel.** Let first the ball of your foot touch the ground, then your toes. Move the other leg slowly forwards, with the heel, ball and toes touching the ground. When moving forwards in slow motion, lift your knee as high as possible and keep your upper body straight.

- **Breathe in as you lift your knee and leg** and breathe out as you bring your leg and foot down. Lengthen your body on the in-breath and move on the out-breath.

- **Try to enjoy every step.** Walk forwards with control and awareness, imagining that your feet are massaging the ground. Walk mindfully for up to 5 minutes.

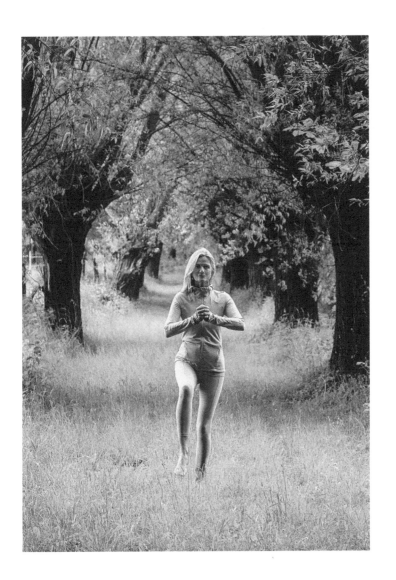

In the traditional *Kinhin*,
walking meditation,
practitioners clasp their
hands in *Shashu*.

Tiptoe Mountain Balance
(Tadasana)

This exercise can be as easy or challenging as you wish. To make it easier, practise without weights. To make it more challenging, move away from the wall, holding your balance without support.

● **Stand against a wall,** with your feet hip-width apart.

● **Bring your arms alongside your body,** holding the weights. Bend your arms and tuck your elbows into your ribcage, like robot arms, creating a right angle, with the weights facing each other.

● **Now, come up onto your tiptoes,** squeeze your glutes and tighten your abs. Breathe out and open your arms out to the side, with your elbows still attached to your ribcage. Breathe in and bring your arms parallel to each other again, with the weights facing each other. Repeat 10 times.

Osteoporosis is not a predestined part of aging; it is treatable, if not preventable.

FURTHER TIPS

● **Calcium is the must-have mineral** that keeps your bones healthy. However, for the calcium to work better, also take vitamin K, vitamin D and the amino acid lysine.[6, 7]

● **Be aware** that there are concerns about the connection between calcium supplements and cardiovascular disease.[8] Therefore, try to get some of your calcium from your food and eat curly kale, broccoli, sardines and oats.

● **Avoid Coca Cola!** The intake of coke (not of other carbonated soft drinks) is associated with low bone mineral density in women. Cola contains caffeine and phosphoric acid (H_3PO_4), which may adversely affect bones.[9]

● **Discuss bisphosphonate medications** (alendronic acid) with your GP. You can either get a yearly injection or take monthly tablets or liquid. Bisphosphonates are a class of drugs that can prevent further loss of bone density, but they are not suitable for everybody, so be aware of the possible side effects, especially to the jaw and teeth.[10]

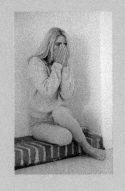

Panic
attacks

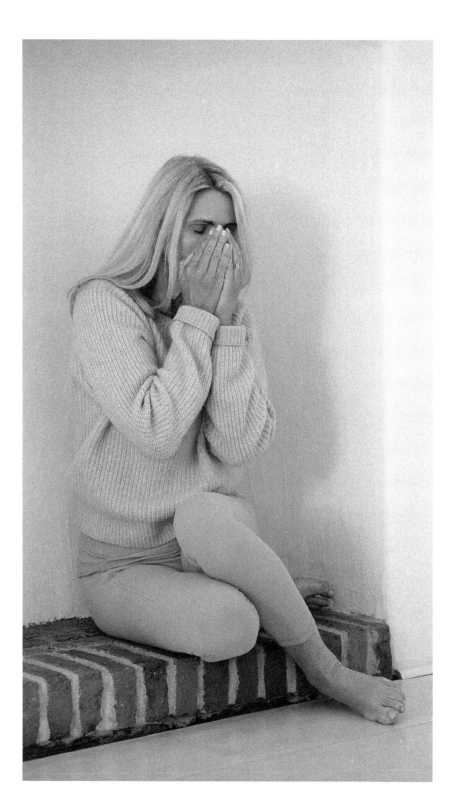

Panic attacks

"I started having panic attacks, and the scariest part was they could be triggered by anything." [1]

Ellie Goulding (Singer)

My first panic attack was in the middle of the night, quite soon after my divorce. I was a single mum lying in bed with my 2 little daughters when, out of nowhere, my heart started pounding like crazy, like it wanted to pop out of my chest. I felt weirdly detached, lightheaded and dizzy, and I could hear my blood passing through my ears. My hands started trembling and my vision became blurry when I looked at my sleeping children.

I felt an overwhelming fear of dying, thinking 'This is what death feels like. I'm going to die, leaving my children alone'. I managed to crawl out of bed and call an ambulance. My heart rate was dangerously high, so my neighbour stayed with my girls, while the paramedics took care of me. At the end of the night, I felt as if all life energy had been sucked out of me.

Every panic attack is scary; the fear is real. I have been there many times, but I have got the right tools now, which help me to manoeuvre through and sometimes prevent panic attacks. These are the tricks and tools I want to share with you.

Most important: during a panic attack try to remind yourself that it is never life-threatening! You are not going to die, and you are not having a heart attack. Constantly reassure yourself that this experience will pass, and you will pull through.

Most panic attacks last 5-20 minutes. Your symptoms will usually be at their worst within 10 minutes. If you experience signs over a longer period, you may be having a second panic attack, or be undergoing other symptoms of anxiety.[2] If you have panic attacks, you are not alone: almost half of the people in Great Britain reported increased feelings of anxiety and fear, due to the uncertainties of Covid and this increase was noted mostly in younger people and women.[3, 4, 5]

You cannot predict when a panic attack will strike, but planning what to do when it happens can help you to feel more in control. Breathing into a paper bag (never into a plastic bag), while covering your mouth and nose can prevent the attack from getting worse. If you do not have a paper bag ready, don't worry; simply breathe into your cupped hands. The idea behind it is to increase your carbon dioxide (CO_2) levels. Do not breathe into a paper bag if you have asthma.

Many people do not realise that CO_2 is actually very important for your body to work properly. When you have a panic attack, it is likely that you will hyperventilate, overbreathe, thereby expelling too much CO_2. Re-breathing the exhaled air can help you to restore the lost gas, and this will make you feel less lightheaded and anxious.

During and after a panic attack try to focus on your breath, doubling your out-breath to your in-breath. This simple technique can help to slow your heart rate, drop your blood pressure and relax your muscles, which is exactly what you need when you are in a panic mode.[6]

If you feel physically drained the day after a panic attack, practise gentle yoga stretches such as the Cat and Cow Stretch (see p.54) or Child's Pose (see p.241). Also, see the Anxiety chapter, (see p.29) and Stress chapter (see p.283).

EXERCISES

Positive Affirmations
(Mantras)

In this exercise, you say positive affirmations – short simple statements – to reassure yourself. Say each one as you breathe in through your nose and out through your mouth, into your cupped hands, which are covering your face.

● **Cup your hands** over your mouth and nose.

● **As you inhale,** say to yourself 'I am not dying', 'I will be fine'. As you exhale, say 'This will soon pass'. You can adapt the affirmations as you wish.

● **Once you feel a bit calmer,** you can drop your hands and continue to breathe in through your nose and out through pursed lips, still repeating your affirmations and synchronising them with your breathing.

● **Continue with your affirmations** until you start doubling your out-breath to your in-breath (see overleaf).

Double the Out-breath

With this simple technique, you can initiate your body into thinking that it is in a relaxed state and that in itself will calm you down.

● **Focus on counting your breath.** Breathe in through your nose for the count of 3 and breathe out through pursed lips for the count of 6, simply doubling your out-breaths to your in-breaths.

● **Continue, in for 3, out for 6, in for 3, out for 6** – there is no holding of the breath, just counting. You may prefer to breathe in for 2, out for 4, or in for 4, out for 8. Do whatever feels most comfortable and calming for you, as long as you are doubling the number of out-breaths to in-breaths.

● **Continue for 3 minutes**.

I use this technique during a panic attack or whenever I feel emotionally overwhelmed.

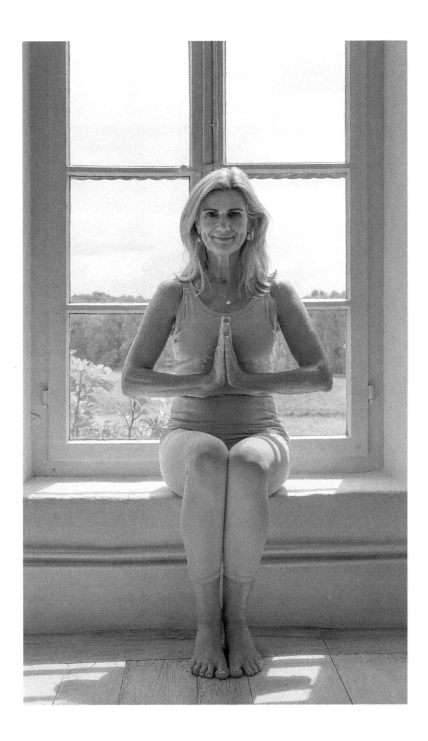

Mindfulness

Panic attacks can cause a feeling of detachment or separation from reality. Practising mindfulness – bringing your awareness back to the present moment – can help to combat a panic attack when it is about to happen, or it can help you to recover from a panic attack that has just happened.[7]

● **Sit down,** preferably on a chair, with a warm drink, with both your feet firmly grounded on the floor.

● **Try to bring all your attention** to the physical sensations you are familiar with, such as the feeling of your feet touching the ground and your bottom touching the chair or floor. Feel the texture of the clothes you are wearing, moving your hands forwards and backwards on your thighs, touching and feeling the fabric. These specific sensations can bring you back to reality and give you something objective to focus on.

● **Now sip your drink.** How does it taste? Is there sweetness or a hint of spice? Whatever the taste, stay with it for a moment longer.

● **Now, rest your hands and look at one familiar thing** in the room. Look at its shape and colour. Just stay focused on that item and silently start to describe it to yourself.

● **Then, close your eyes,** if it feels safe to do so, and listen. Is there anything you can hear? Maybe the soft snoring sound of your own breath? Stay with your breath for a moment, listening to each in- and-out-breath sounding a bit like ocean waves. If you do not like to listen to your breath, play a song you normally enjoy and find calming.

● **Finally, move your awareness to your nose** and smell the scent in the room. If you have any bergamot or lavender oils, dilute a few drops in a glass of warm water. Bring the cup close to your nose and smell the deliciously relaxing essential oils. Do not drink it, just smell it. Some oils have a really calming effect that can help to reduce anxiety, stress or panic.[8]

Practising mindfulness – bringing your awareness back to the present moment – can help to combat a panic attack or calm you afterwards.

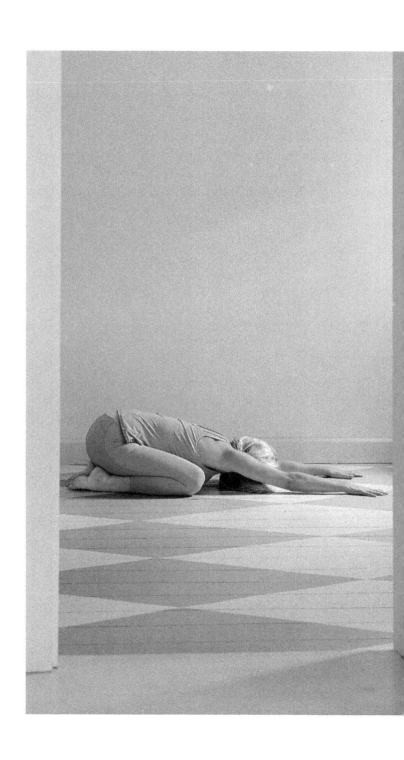

Child's Pose (Balasana)

This gentle, restorative yoga posture can help you to recover from a panic attack. If your head cannot reach the floor, rest it on a yoga brick. If your bottom cannot reach your heels, place a folded blanket behind your knees.

● **Kneel on the floor and sit on your heels,** separating your knees about as wide as your hips. If your body is rather hypermobile and flexible, bring your knees closer together. If your body feels rather stiff, bring your knees more than hip-width apart.

● **Exhale and relax your upper body** in-between or onto your thighs. Broaden your tailbone and lengthen it away from the back of your pelvis. Keep your arms either alongside your upper body or stretch them out in front of you – whatever feels most comfortable.

● **Let your forehead rest on the floor** and breathe deeply, focusing on a long out-breath and the sensation of your body touching the ground.

● **Stay in the pose** for several minutes.

FURTHER TIPS

● **Vitamin B12 and magnesium** are safe remedies that appear to help with panic and anxiety.[9, 10]

● **Use essential oils.** Put a few drops of bergamot oil, sage or lavender into a bowl of warm water and the deliciously uplifting scent will fill the room. If you prefer something warmer and spicy, use frankincense and sandalwood.[11] As well as enjoying the scents, treat yourself to an aromatherapy massage or use the oils for self-massage.

● **Consider counselling or CBT** (cognitive behavioural therapy). It can be so helpful to talk to someone about your worries and fears and learn how to let go of them.[12]

● **Ask your GP about escitalopram,** which is a type of anti-depressant known as a selective serotonin reuptake inhibitor (SSRI). It is supposed to help with panic attacks.[13]

I've been taking it for several years now and, even though it is the lowest possible dose of 5mg, it seems to work.

● **If you witness someone** having a panic attack, react calmly, and be reassuring and understanding.

● **For support with panic attacks,** contact No Panic, everyday 10am-10pm Helpline number (UK) 0300 772 9844. Youth Line 0333 772 2644. Or contact the Mind helpline to talk about your panic attacks and anxiety. info@mind.org.uk Infoline: (UK) 0300 123 3393 It is open 9am to 6pm, Monday to Friday (except for bank holidays).

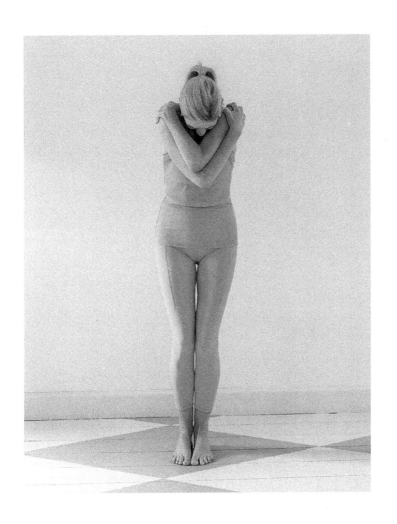

Constantly reassure yourself
that this experience
will pass and you will
pull through.

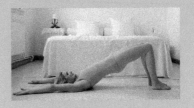

Queefs

I regularly practise exercises that strengthen my pelvic floor muscles and bladder function, preventing queefing and improving our sex life.

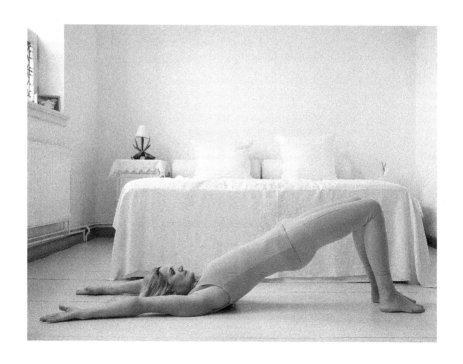

Queefs

"They never ever taught us that we are capable of queefing ..." [1]

Tiffany Haddish (Actress)

I was once young and in love and wanted to sleep with my boyfriend, but all I can remember is that my body produced kind of embarrassing sounds during sex. This was not something I expected or was able to control.

Queefing is the audible release of air from the vagina, otherwise known as fanny farts. It is completely natural, considering that the vagina isn't a straight tube and air can easily get trapped in there during sex. Queefing can happen during yoga as well, especially when you are transitioning from one pose into another. Before you know it, you have expelled the tiniest 'poof', which if it happens in a packed yoga class can be a bit awkward. Certain yoga exercises can help you to reduce vagina farts while others can set them off. Try to avoid poses that put pressure on your pelvic area and shoulder, such as shoulder or head stands.

During sex you can practise positions that minimise the amount of air getting into your vagina - the missionary position being the safest. If you prefer more variety in your sex life, such as doggy style or inverted missionary with the woman on top, you will be automatically more prone to queefing.

Personally, I no longer allow a silly sound to affect my sex life, but I am not keen on queefing in front of my yoga class. Therefore, I regularly practise exercises that strengthen my pelvic floor muscles and bladder function, preventing queefing and improving my sex life.

EXERCISES

Root Lock (Mula Bandha)

Mula Bandha is a great tool to improve your sex life (see Sex chapter, p.265) and to prevent any unwanted noises.

Caution: Do not practise this exercise if you have intestinal ulcers, a hernia, high blood pressure, heart disease, glaucoma or if you are pregnant or menstruating.

● **Sit on a chair or on the floor,** with your spine straight and your eyes closed. Bring awareness to the base of your spine and your genitals.

● **Try tightening and relaxing the muscle fibres at the front,** around your vagina. Continue this for a while and then start tightening and relaxing the muscles around your anus. The whole action should feel as though you are trying to stop passing urine and stop passing wind at the same time.

● **Continue squeezing and releasing,** then relax and focus on a few in- and out-breaths through your nostrils, not your mouth.

● **Then after your next out-breath,** close both your nostrils (with your index finger and thumb) and do the same action as if you are inhaling through your nostrils, but without breathing in (not even through your mouth).

● **While pretending to breathe in,** try to lift all the muscles around the vagina and anus upwards. Hold them tight and then release as you breathe out.

● **Practise the tightening and lifting** of the sphincter, anal and pelvic floor muscles, while standing in a queue, sitting at your desk or on public transport. Nobody will notice! This regular training can prevent queefing and incontinence, and enhance your sexual experiences.

Bridge Pose (Dvi Pada Pitham)

Moving on the out-breath can reduce the amount of air your body takes in, thereby reducing the possibility of queefing.

● **Lie on your back** and bend your legs.

● **Keep your feet and knees parallel** to each other, hip-width apart.

● **Position your arms by your side** with your palms facing downwards.

● **Breathe in** through your nose and relax.

● **Now, breathe out,** and lift your hips and back while squeezing your pelvic floor muscles. Hold the bridge position, breathing in. Breathe out and release your spine back down. Repeat 10 times.

● **For more of a challenge,** remain in the Bridge Pose for a little bit longer, while trying to incorporate the Root Lock (see opposite page).

Sitting Cow
(Upavistha Bitilasana Marjaryasana)

You can practise this exercise with or without breath retention, but it is more effective if you can hold your breath.

Caution: Do not hold your breath if you are pregnant, or if you have untreated high blood pressure or asthma. Instead, try to breathe in and out through your nose slowly.

- **Sit on the floor,** with your legs bent and your feet hip-width apart. Place your hands on the outside of your knees. As you inhale, roll forwards on your sitting bones, lift your chest and gently arch your spine.

- **As you exhale,** push your pelvis slightly forwards. Round first your lower back, then the middle part and finally the upper part of your back and neck, straightening your arms.

- **Retain your breath** after the out-breath, while holding the position, until you feel that you are running out of oxygen.

- **Then, slowly release** first your deep abdominal muscles, before you breathe in again, coming back up into the neutral position. If you try to breathe in without releasing your muscles first, you will start coughing. Take a normal in-breath and out-breath before you start another round.

- **Repeat** 10 times.

- **To finish,** roll all the way down onto the floor and relax.

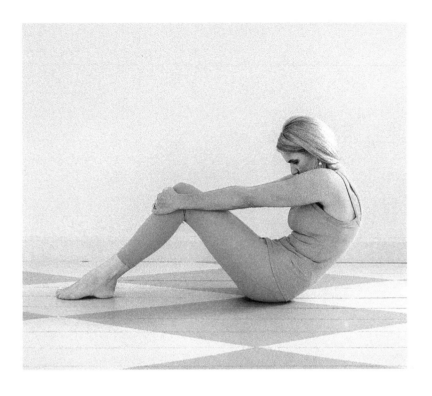

FURTHER TIPS

● **Use a tampon,** even when you are not menstruating, just for the duration of the yoga class, because then no air can be expelled through your vagina.

● **Try sitting backwards on the toilet** when you pee (aka straddling the seat facing the back of the toilet). This is supposed to open your vaginal canal and can help to release some of the trapped air in your vagina.

● **Avoid fast, jackhammer-style sex** so that less air will be trapped in your vagina.

● **Remember, fanny farts are a natural bodily function** and nothing to be embarrassed about.

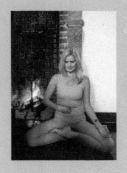

Reflux

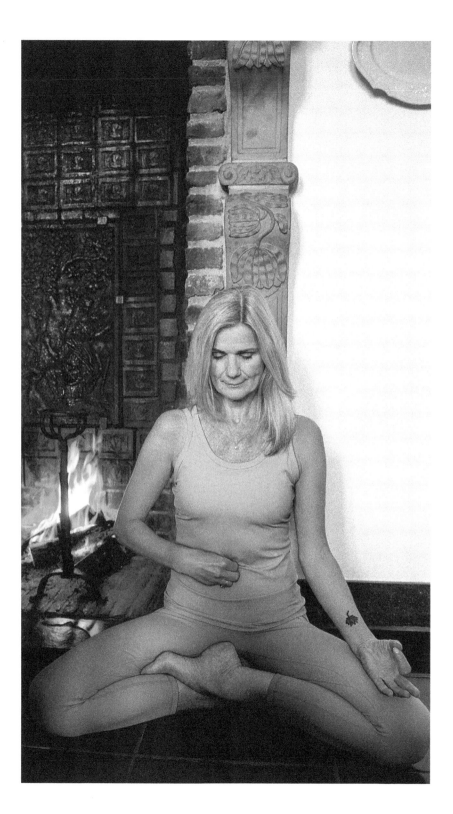

Reflux

"I would like to find a stew that will give me heartburn immediately, instead of at 3 o'clock in the morning." [1]

John Barrymore (Actor)

My first husband had an affair with one of my best friends and the impact of this double betrayal triggered a massive overflow of acidity in my body, which affected my tummy and my vocal cords. I even lost my voice for weeks. I didn't know how to articulate my feelings anymore. I felt hurt, humiliated and incredibly sad.

Eventually, of course, I was able to speak again. My husband left me and our kids to be with his new girlfriend, but the acid reflux, commonly known as heartburn, stuck with me, continuing to cause problems. Since then, I have learned to manage my condition and have even been able to reduce my medication. Stress triggered the heartburn in the first place, but it was my disposition (see overleaf) that enabled it over the years.

Reflux affects up to 25% of UK adults. It can be annoying, frustrating and downright painful to deal with. Although occasional acid reflux cannot kill you, it can substantially affect your quality of life and, if left untreated, can increase your risk of developing oesophageal cancer.[2, 3]

It is hard to eliminate acid reflux, but there are a few things you can do. From a yogic perspective, it is most important to give yourself time to heal and to balance your inner fire.

Yoga's sister science *Ayurveda*, the Indian science of life and health, can help you to heal by finding the right inner balance. *Ayurveda* distinguishes between three different types of constitutions, called *Doshas*: *Vata* (air), *Kapha* (earth) and *Pitta* (fire). They all represent various qualities that apply not only to your physical body, but also to your mind and emotions. Although most of us are a combination of all 3 *Doshas*, 1 might be more dominant. To determine your *Doshic* type see page 330 or consult an Ayurvedic practitioner.

Once you know your *Dosha* type, you can follow the recommendations, including adjusting your diet and the way you exercise yoga. For example: a *Pitta* type, who has too much 'fire' in comparison to the other elements, tends to have a strong drive and likes a challenging and competitive environment. Their chosen yoga routine is often fast and powerful, such as *Ashtanga*, but what they probably should practise instead is something more restorative, such as *Yin Yoga*, or a static yoga, such as *Iyengar*.

Over the years, I have often seen that the yoga style or exercises someone prefers are not necessarily the ones they need. Here is an example: I lack *Kapha* and have lots of *Vata* and *Pitta*. Therefore, I benefit from simple grounding exercises rather than inversions, which I love. The same goes for food: I prefer spicy and salty raw food but, according to my constitution, I should cook my vegetables and start the day with a warm porridge and oat milk. It is more than just changing your food from acidic to alkaline because once you eat and practise according to and in harmony with your *Doshic* constitution, your reflux should lessen and you can reduce or even stop any medication.

The yoga postures that I recommend in this chapter should be practised slowly and in harmony with your breath. Think healing, rather than firing up your system. Start with *Nadi Shodhana Pranayama*, the Alternate Nostril Breathing that can balance your system, restoring equilibrium. The Mountain Pose is a good posture to begin with and from there you can move into a standing backbend or side bend. Just be aware that bending forwards and inversions are not recommended when your reflux is acute.

Furthermore, I suggest that you discover the kind and gentle warrior within you. The Warrior II Pose can help to release tension in your ribcage and abdomen, supporting your healing process. Finally, try my Love Your Belly Breath, a tapping and breathing exercise that can calm down, rather than ignite, your inner fire. Consider your belly to be like your second brain. You will feel it there first when you are happy or in danger. Tapping your belly button can help you to reconnect with where you come from – your family history, your past. And sometimes re-establishing this relationship is important to enable you to move forwards without any bitterness or aggression towards yourself or others.

Nurture your inner fire, passion and willpower, but don't allow the fire to take over.

EXERCISES

Alternate Nostril Breathing
(Nadi Shodhana Pranayama)

This relaxing breathing exercise can help to balance the right and left sides of your brain. Before you start, try to work out which of your nostrils feels more blocked or is more open. After the exercise, you might notice that the flow of breath has changed, and both your nostrils feel open.

The two fingers you will use in this hand action (*Vishnu Mudra*) are your thumb (representing the element of fire) and your ring finger (representing the earth).

Caution: Those suffering with high blood pressure, heart disease or peptic ulcers should never hold their breath.

● **You may want to blow your nose** before you begin.

● **Sit comfortably on the floor,** using a yoga block if it helps, or on the edge of a chair. Roll your shoulders up, back and down. Repeat a couple of times.

● **Ground yourself** through an awareness of your sitting bones touching the floor, block or chair. Lift your chest and heart, keeping your spine as straight as possible.

● **Place your right hand in front of your face,** with your arm vertical in front of your chest. If you wish, your elbow can be supported by your other hand, without restricting your chest.

- **Close your right nostril with your right thumb** and inhale deeply through your left nostril. At the peak of your inhalation, close both your nostrils, by pressing your ring finger against your left nostril. Then lift your thumb and breathe out slowly through your right nostril.

- **After a full exhalation,** inhale through the right nostril, close both nostrils again, then breathe out through your left nostril. Continue Alternate Nostril Breathing for up to 3 minutes.

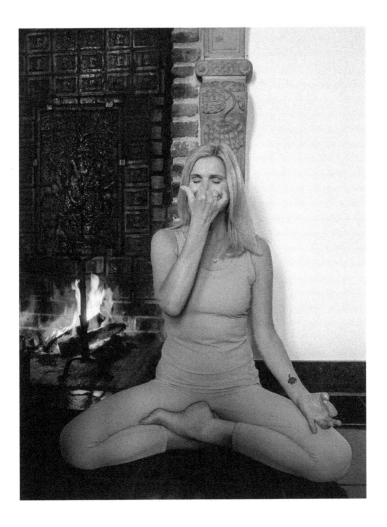

Mountain Pose (Tadasana)

This grounding pose helps you to improve your posture, potentially reducing pressure on your oesophagus, which is helpful when you have reflux.

- **Stand with your bare feet hip-width apart**. Spread your toes apart and lift them all up (yes, even the little ones). Bring them down again, pressing your big toes into the floor. Feel how this helps you to lift your inner thigh muscles and kneecaps.

- **Now, squeeze your bottom a bit** to position your pelvis and lengthen your neck away from your shoulders, dropping your shoulder blades down towards your tailbone. You can close your eyes, if you wish.

- **Gently shift your whole body** (keeping it as straight as a plank) forwards and back without taking your heels or toes off the floor. Move forwards and back until you find your centre.

- **Inhale deeply** and lift both your arms over your head, palms facing each other. Exhale gently and release your arms to shoulder height, palms facing downwards.

- **Count to 6 as you breathe in through your nose,** lifting your arms. Breathe out to the count of 6 through your mouth, releasing your arms.

- **Now, bend your legs as you release your arms** and straighten your legs as you lift them, keeping your knees and breath soft. Keep your upper body straight when bending your legs.

- **Repeat** as many times as you like.

Warrior II (Virabhadrasana II)

Like the Mountain Pose, Warrior II is believed to aid digestion and reduce the pressure on the oesophagus, therefore preventing reflux symptoms.

● **Place your hands on your hips**, bend your legs and silently jump them apart, using your core strength. Turn your right foot 90 degrees outwards and your left foot slightly inwards.

● **Lift your arms out to the side** at shoulder height with your palms facing downwards. Exhale and bend your right knee to a 90-degree angle. Keep pressing into your left heel and make sure that you keep your upper body straight, not leaning towards the right.

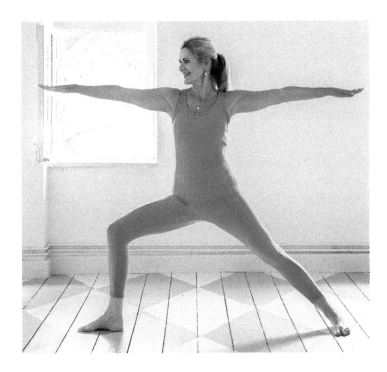

● **Drop your shoulder blades down,** relax your neck and jaw, and smile. Look over to your right hand, focusing on your middle finger for a moment. Stay in this pose for a couple of slow in-breaths through your nose and out-breaths through your nose or mouth. Feel how you expand your ribcage with each in-breath, creating space around your breastbone. This tends to be the place where you can feel most pain when suffering from acid reflux.

● **Be kind to yourself** and do not force yourself to hold the posture longer than you want. Repeat on the other side.

Love Your Belly Breath

This mindful breathing and tapping exercise focuses on your belly button and the *Manipura Chakra* (see p.329), the seat of willpower and strength. Each finger represents an element and bringing them together into *Mukula Mudra* can focus energy where healing is required.

● **Sit on the floor** or on the edge of a chair with your spine straight and your belly relaxed and soft. If you are right-handed, use your left hand first and vice versa.

● **Bring all 5 fingertips of one hand together** into the shape of a beak, the *Mukula Mudra*, then direct them towards your belly button.

● **Remind yourself to keep your belly soft,** while gently tapping your fingertips against your belly button. Keep tapping your belly button for approximately 1 minute.

● **Repeat the above** with the other hand for 1 minute.

● **Then, alternate the tapping** with both your hands.

● **To finish,** shake out your hands and relax.

FURTHER TIPS

● **Start each day** by drinking a mug of warm lemon water with fresh ginger and a bit of manuka honey. Even though lemon is acidic, once inside your body it transforms to be alkaline. Drinking at least 2 litres of still water (no carbonated beverages) over the day can neutralise stomach acidity.

● **Eat regular, small meals.** The higher the volume of food in your stomach, the more chance there is of it 'splashing' up and into your oesophagus.

● **Eat extremely slowly** to help with your digestion (constipation can trigger reflux), and to feel less bloated (flatulence can be a side effect of heartburn).

● **Eat lots of dark-green vegetables** to help create a more alkaline environment in your body. If you do not like to eat vegetables, cook them then blend them to use in a soup or as pasta sauce.

● **Cut out alcohol,** coffee and red meat. I know that sounds a bit drastic, but it can be a game changer.[4, 5]

● **Elevate the head of your bed** a couple of inches to prevent the acidity from getting into your oesophagus while sleeping and try to sleep on your left side.

● **PPIs** (proton pump inhibitors) are the most powerful medications for relieving heartburn. However, do not rely on them forever. Prolonged use of PPIs is a risk factor for a variety of diseases, including osteoporosis and anaemia due to lack of absorption of calcium, iron and vitamins.[6]

● **If you opt for anti-reflux surgery** (fundoplication), be aware that it is quite an invasive operation (even with keyhole, there is up to 6 weeks of recovery) and there is no guarantee that it will work.

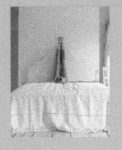

Sex

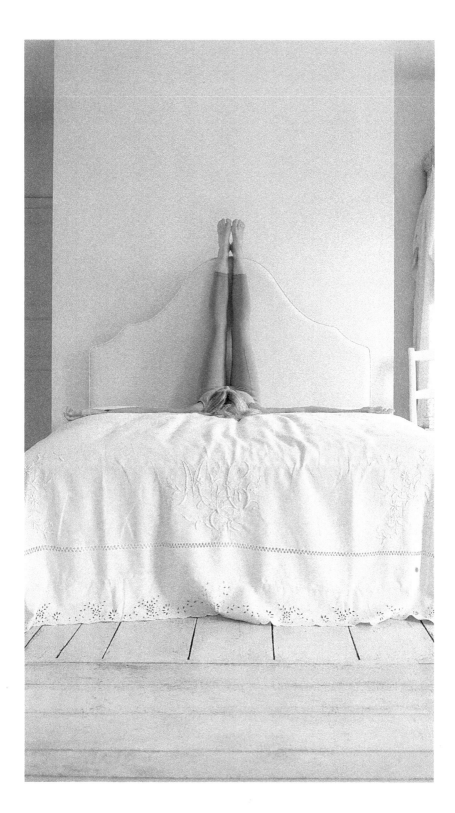

Sex

"Good sex is like good bridge. If you don't have a good partner, you'd better have a good hand." [1]

Mae West (Actress)

One of the many reasons why my husband and I are still together is because we enjoy having sex with each other. After more than 27 years, I still like to smell and touch his skin and make love to him. However, we don't have sex as often as we used to and it sometimes lacks a bit of spontaneity and requires strategic planning: 'Be careful, my left shoulder hurts', or 'Remember, you have to be on top because of my back'. I feel the urge to talk before having sex and my husband likes to fall asleep immediately after. I don't mind not having sex for weeks, whereas such a gap makes my husband feel grumpy and neglected. These differences will probably never change, but one thing is certain: whenever we have had sex, we tend to be much more tolerant towards each other … at least for a couple of hours.

Despite feeling happier because of sex, initiating it in a long-term relationship can be hard work, requiring creativity, patience and a sense of humour. Even when a couple is having sex regularly, it is common for one partner to want more sex, while the other might think it is the quality, not the quantity, that counts. The truth probably lies somewhere in the middle. Perhaps sex is like money – none or too little is bad, but too much is not necessarily better.[2]

So, how many times have you had sex in the past month? I know this tends to be a sensitive topic, with at least half of the

British population preferring not to discuss their sex life and approximately 3 in 10 Brits being sexually inactive. This lack of activity is influenced by physical and emotional experiences, various lifestyles, relationship status and it seems that the older we get, the less interested we are in having sex.[3]

Regardless of our sexual orientation or preferences, sexual intercourse, which ranges from penetration, oral sex, or any other activity culminating in orgasm, reaps many health benefits. It can unleash all kind of chemical compounds into our brain, making us feel better, both mentally and physically. Regular sex can improve our memory and sleep, strengthen our heart, reduce the risk of prostate cancer, tone our pelvic floor muscles and bladder, decrease feelings of stress and pain, support our immune system and, finally, sex can prolong our life expectancy![4, 5]

Therefore, despite a possible lack of interest, old age, shape or size, try to enjoy your sexuality. Do not just ignore it because life may be getting in the way.

Yoga certainly can improve your sex life. A regular yoga practice can help you to feel more confident and relaxed in your own body. It can reactivate your desire, and appears to improve arousal, lubrication, orgasm and satisfaction. Furthermore, yoga helps you to become more attuned to the needs and feelings of others, which can make you a better, more attentive, sexual partner.[6, 7]

You have probably heard of *Tantra Yoga* and Tantric sex – the singer Sting once famously mentioned it in an interview. *Tantra Yoga* used to be a preferred practice in ancient India for enhanced sexual pleasure and Tantric sex revolves around practices that focus on creating a deep, intimate connection. During Tantric sex, the aim is to be present in the moment, in a meditative state, to achieve a sensual and fulfilling sexual

The benefits of regular sex

These benefits are for all genders, but associated with specifically penile-vaginal intercourse.

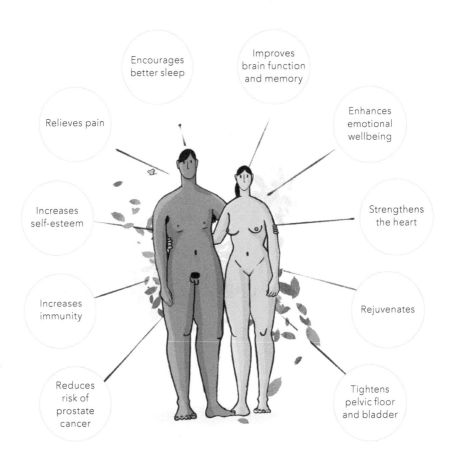

Encourages better sleep

Improves brain function and memory

Relieves pain

Enhances emotional wellbeing

Increases self-esteem

Strengthens the heart

Increases immunity

Rejuvenates

Reduces risk of prostate cancer

Tightens pelvic floor and bladder

experience. Then, when you reach your climax, you are completely absorbed in the present, entering timelessness for a couple of seconds and maybe that's the reason why the French call an orgasm *'La petite mort'*, 'the little death'.

Tantra Yoga, just like any other form of *Hatha Yoga*, can include the powerful combination of exercise (*Asana*), symbolic gestures (*Mudra*), energy locks (*Bandhas*) and energy centres (*Chakras*). There are thousands of chakras throughout your body, but yoga focuses on the 7 main ones (see p.328).

Bandhas are locks that work on a physical and spiritual level (see Queefs chapter, p.245 and Fat Belly chapter, p.87). There are three *bandhas*, but in this chapter we concentrate on the so-called Root Lock, the *Mula Bandha*. This bandha can be a powerful tool when performing sexual intercourse. In men, it can help with erectile function and ejaculation; in women, the squeezing and tightening of the pelvic floor muscles can enhance arousal and sexual sensation.

Engaging the pelvic floor muscles before and during sex can intensify the sexual encounter for all parties involved. Additionally, the more sex you practise, the stronger your pelvic floor muscles will become and the stronger the pelvic floor, the more you will be able to enjoy and perform sex. Sounds simple, right? So, how can you find and train these all-important muscles? They are hidden deep in your lower abdomen where they form a large sling, like a hammock, stretching from side to side across your pelvic floor, attached to the pubic bone at the front and the tailbone at the back. It requires a bit of patience and time to locate them properly.

So, let's start with finding and working the deepest pelvic floor muscle, which is called the *levator ani* and that means - no joke, or pun intended, raise the bottom.

EXERCISES

Perineum Contractions
(Mula Bandha)

Mula Bandha can lead to increased sensitivity and more intense and satisfying orgasms. Practise the squeezing and lifting of your pelvic floor muscles daily for a couple of minutes. After a while, you can start using this technique during intercourse.

● **Sit comfortably,** on the edge of a chair is preferable, and relax with your spine straight and your hands on your thighs.

● **Close your eyes** and bring your awareness to your pelvis, seat of the *Muladhara Chakra* (see p.329), the energy centre located in your perineum, the space between the anus and scrotum and between the anus and vulva.

● **Start by tightening and relaxing** just the muscle fibres in the front, around your penis or vagina (*Vajroli/Sahajoli Mudra*) - this action can feel as though you are trying to stop yourself from peeing. Continue to breathe normally while clenching and relaxing your muscles.

● **Next, start to tighten** the muscles around your anus (*Ashwini Mudra*). This action can feel as though you are trying to stop yourself from passing wind. Continue the squeezing and letting go of these muscles a couple of times.

● **Then, squeeze *all* the muscles**, at the front and the back and it can feel as if you are trying to stop passing urine and wind at the same time. While maintaining the contraction, continue to breathe slowly and smoothly.

● **In addition, while contracting the muscles,** try to pull them up towards your belly. Imagine a lift going up to the first, second and third floor, which is around the height of your navel. Hold tight for a couple of seconds and then release the muscles again while breathing out.

● **Take a deep breath in** and repeat the clenching, lifting and holding of the muscles, then release the lock with your out-breath. Repeat 10 more times.

● **Once the contraction can be held for longer** and without affecting your breath, you will be able to incorporate the lock during sex.

The possible firmer grip
around the penis can be
a game-changer for
all parties involved.

Hip Circling

This exercise is from *Kundalini Yoga*, which is believed to help to attain a satisfying sex life. The hip circling can unleash and increase your sexual desire and energy, affecting the *Swadhisthana Chakra* (see p.329), your sacral energy centre. It is the second lowest chakra and the seat of your emotions, sexual energy and creativity.

● **Sit down in any cross-legged position.** Keep your hands on your knees and bring awareness to your pelvis. With your eyes closed or open, begin to circle your hips clockwise while keeping your upper body straight. Make sure that the movement comes from your pelvis and not from your waist or shoulders.

● **Keep moving your hips** in small and compressed circles for approximately 1–2 minutes.

● **Stay in the rhythm,** focusing on the area around the base of your spine and your perineum.

Goddess Pose
(Utkata Konasana)

This exercise reminds me of the *Haka*, the ceremonial dance of the *Maori* people, used by the All-Blacks Rugby team. The full Goddess Pose (see photo, p.279) is just as impressive. The goddess can stimulate your sexual organs, activate your sacral chakra, strengthen your pelvic floor and open your hips.

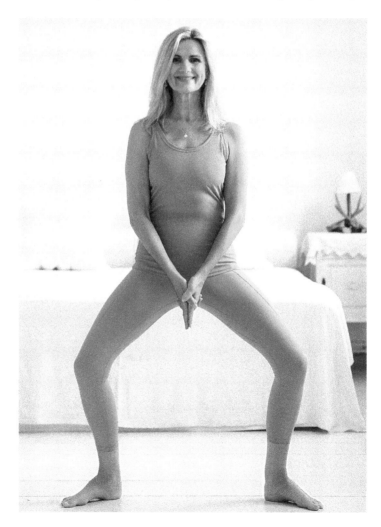

Caution: Do not hold your breath if you are pregnant, or if you have any heart issues, high blood pressure or glaucoma.

● **Stand and silently jump your legs apart.** Turn your feet slightly outwards, bend both your legs, and bring your hands together in front of your lower abdomen, extending your index fingers downwards into *Kali Mudra*. Men are supposed to press both their thumbs together, while women keep the right thumb between the left thumb and index finger.

● **Now, gently rock from side to side.** Make sure that your upper body remains as straight as possible, while your legs are bent, with your tailbone swinging from side to side. Eventually, stop moving and remain in the centre with your legs bent.

● **Slightly tilt your pelvis forwards** and squeeze the sphincter, the vaginal and anal muscles, lifting them all up towards your navel, performing the *Mula Bandha* (see p.271) on your in-breath. Hold your breath for a few seconds, then release the muscles with your out-breath. Straighten your legs and relax for a moment.

● **Bend your legs again** and take your arms out to the side, at shoulder height, with your index finger and thumb touching (*Chin Mudra*). Create right angles with your upper and lower arms and your legs. Now, lift first the right heel, then the left and eventually both heels off the floor.

● **Breathe in and tilt your pelvis slightly forwards,** while squeezing and lifting your pelvic floor muscles. Hold your breath, while staying in the pose with your upper body as straight as possible. Breathe out, straighten your legs, drop your heels and release your arms. Repeat once more.

Yogic Gazing (Trataka)

To promote better communication and trust, practise Yogic Gazing with a partner. Some couples like to do it before they have sex because it can help to create more intimacy. Alternatively, do this exercise alone, in front of a mirror. Take off your glasses if you are short-sighted and be aware that the exercise might not work while wearing contact lenses.

● **Kneel, with your bottom resting on your heels** if possible. Use a cushion in-between your heels and bottom to make it more comfortable or, alternatively, sit on a chair. Sit opposite your partner, with your knees touching. Your eyes need to be at the same level, so raise your bottom if you need to.

● **Look at your partner (or yourself in the mirror) and smile,** without talking. After a few giggles, notice that you can see your own reflection in your partner's eyes. Focus on just one eye. Imagine that you are sinking into your partner's (or your own) pupil, and this can feel like diving into a beautiful calm lake.

● **When your eyes start watering** and you need to blink, gently close your eyes for a moment. Then re-open your eyes and gaze at your partner's eye, or your own, again. The more relaxed you are, the less likely you will need to blink.

● **Next time you close your eyes,** visualise your partner's eye in your inner eye. When this image begins to fade, open your eyes again and look at the real eye. Continue this process of gazing outwards and inwards as often as you like. This can go on for seconds, minutes or hours, it is up to you. Once you want to finish the exercise, just keep your eyes closed.

● **After this experience** you will probably feel quite connected and chatty; any kind of reaction is fine. My husband just looked at me a bit clueless and instantly asked, 'And? Will we have sex now?' and that made me laugh.

Father-Mother (Yab-Yum)

This classic seated Tantric sex position can align your chakras with your partner's and allows you to breathe in harmony with each other. This exercise, as well as all the others in this chapter, is for couples of all orientations. In a same-sex relationship, which polarity you choose depends on you. Masculine and feminine are simply 2 parts of a whole and you choose which you sense is your polarity.[8]

Father-Mother can be done fully clothed or naked and before, during or instead of sex.

● **One person, usually the larger person,** sits cross-legged. The other person then sits on their partner's thighs with their ankles crossed behind their partner's back. Alternatively, both of you keep your legs extended.

● **With your foreheads touching** (*Ajna Chakra*), place your arms comfortably around each other. Now, close your eyes and focus on your breath and your partner's breath as the main point of your connection.

● **Inhale together,** pause together, exhale together and pause again. Connect directly with your partner's breath and enjoy the warmth and energy coming from you and your partner. Stay in this embrace for as long as you both like.

You are now united as 2 complementary aspects in the union of masculine and feminine, of *Yab-Yum*.

If you prefer lying down to sitting, then try this modification of *Yab-Yum*. In this Tantric exercise, you are snuggled up in a spooning position, lying on your left sides. The (larger) partner lying at the back will want to slip their arm under their partner's neck, supporting their own head with a cushion. Their right hand can rest on their partner's heart (*Anahata Chakra*) or the left breast. Both partners try to line up their main energy centres, the chakras.

● **While lying comfortably,** notice your partner's breath and begin to synchronise your breath: take a deep breath in together, pause together and breathe out together, pausing again. You are not holding your breath, just noticing brief pauses between each in- and out-breath.

● **Once both your breaths seem to merge,** you can feel the energy effortlessly flowing, allowing both of you to unite completely, feeling as one being in a single wholeness in this moment. This can be a moment of sheer bliss, your bodies close together, breathing in harmony with each other.

● **Stay for as long as you like in this position,** simply enjoying the union.

● **When it is time to let go,** gently release and physically move away from each other, while turning your faces towards each other, smiling.

● **Next time you repeat the exercise,** change position with the larger person lying at the front.

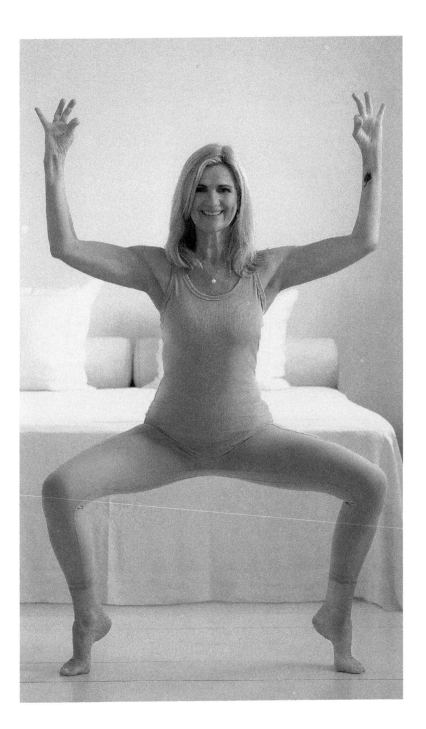

FURTHER TIPS

● **Stay curious:** explore new techniques, sex toys and different positions in various places at unusual times. Alternatively, use your own imagination – this can be a great stimulant for you and your partner.

● **Get sweaty by exercising** before you have sex – it can make it easier for you to get aroused.[9]

● **In case you are single** with no partner in sight, you can still enjoy pleasuring yourself regularly. Invest in a vibrator. Most of them are very handy and discreet, such as the Quiet G-spot Petite Rabbit. If you are more adventurous, buy the potent Rampant Rabbit and discover what arouses you by experimenting with different speeds and several vibration patterns.

● **There is more to the clitoris than meets the eye:** most people think that the clitoris is a small pleasure zone tucked inside the vulva (vulva is outside, vagina inside), but it extends well into the pelvis and has a concentration of lots of nerve endings, more than the head of the penis.

● **Curious men** could try out a prostate massager, stimulating the male 'G-spot' and enhancing the intensity of the orgasm.

● **Choose the right perfume** or aftershave. Some scents can calm or excite us and play an important part in physical attraction. The aromatic oils that are supposed to have aphrodisiac qualities are the sweeter flavours of vanilla, rose, jasmine, patchouli and ylang-ylang.

- **Try vabbing,** using your vaginal fluid as perfume, to attract the opposite sex. At the heart of vabbing is the concept of pheromones, chemicals secreted outside the body, used for signalling between members of the same species.[10]

- **Look into supplements. L-arginine and yohimbine** can help to improve blood circulation and so benefit those who suffer from sexual dysfunction or a low libido.[11] Ashwagandha is thought to improve sexual and psychological wellbeing.[12] Always consult your GP before taking supplements.

Try to see the funny side of sex. The person with whom you can enjoy sex and laughter is a keeper!

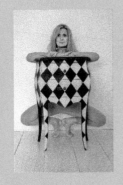

Stress

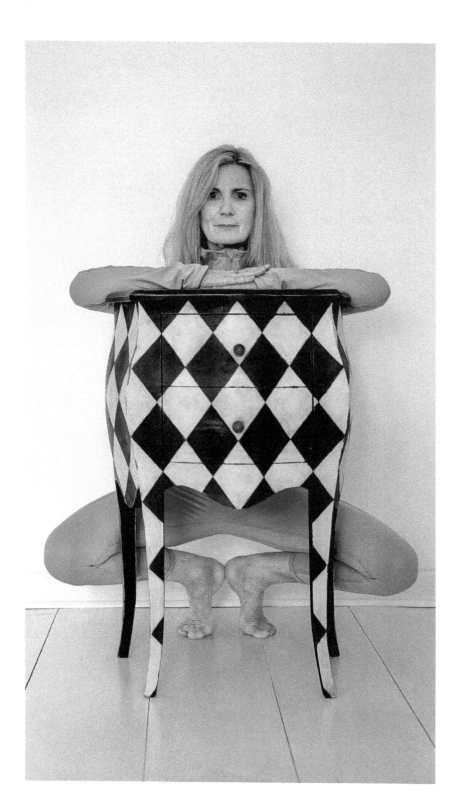

Stress

"It's not stress that kills us; it is our reaction to it" [1]

Hans Selye (Endocrinologist)

When stressed, my skin starts itching, my tummy makes weird noises, and I can no longer reflect properly. I retreat to black-and-white thinking, with my brain focusing on the one mindset that makes me feel most safe: the 'I am right, and you are wrong' perspective. For example, if I am late for work and cannot find my keys, instead of recalling my last whereabouts, I start shouting questions and blaming others for moving my keys, which then, of course, causes more stress and tension.

On the other hand, I do hold the capacity to thrive on stress. For example, when I need to give an important presentation I love the exhilarating feeling of all the stress hormones rushing through my system, enabling me to deliver my best possible performance. I feel pressure, but at the same time I am excited and highly motivated, riding on a wave of positive stress, instead of drowning in it.

Furthermore, I believe that it was stress that helped me to cope with a lot of things when I was a teenager. I had to be switched on all the time, taking on far more responsibilities than any child should have to. I wanted to get out and find my own path. Without stress I would not have managed to succeed in that. However, once I felt safe, my body was so used to all the cortisol and adrenaline that, without it, I felt a bit like a junkie without drugs. I was so accustomed to feeling stressed that I could not relax. This was the time when I found yoga. I was still a teenager and yoga seemed to offer everything I lacked: a calm, reflective, reliable routine – a haven amidst all the chaos. And, 50 years later, yoga still helps me to turn bad stress into good stress and to feel alive without tension and hassle.

Everyone should consider trying yoga when they are dealing with life's pressures because the impact of long-term stress can be devastating to your health. The stress hormone cortisol can, over the long term, suppress the immune system, increasing blood pressure and sugar levels, and decreasing the libido. Persistent surges of adrenaline can damage blood vessels, elevating the risk of a heart attack or stroke. Also, long-term stress can fast-track biological aging and result in anxiety and depression.[2] A UK survey found that the most common causes of stress were work (79%), money (60%) and family (48%).[3, 4]

So, what exactly can yoga do to prevent long-term stress and change your response towards it?[5] Firstly, get to know your vagus nerve, the longest nerve in your body, which connects your brain to many important organs, including the gut, stomach, heart and lungs. By stimulating the vagus nerve, you can send a message to your body that it is time to relax and de-stress (see Anxiety chapter, p.29).

Furthermore, I suggest that you have a look at Kriyas, which are so-called cleansing exercises. They can help you to get rid of negative emotions that trigger stress (see Anger chapter, p15).

Kriyas can help to shift the balance from the sympathetic nervous system, the 'fight or flight' response, to the parasympathetic system, the 'rest and digest' response. Combining a *Kriya* with a *Mantra*, a positive affirmation, can be powerful and there is some evidence that *Mantra* meditation can improve your mental health and stress response.[6]

Thousands of years ago, yoga's initial goal was to conquer fear of death and to prepare the body for meditation, because a calm mind does not get stressed easily. This goal of meditation is consistent with a more recent technique, which is called Progressive Muscle Relaxation, PMR. Relaxation techniques such as PMR can reverse your stress response, calming your mind, reducing body tension through systematically squeezing and then releasing isolated muscle groups.[7]

Moreover, try *Savitri* breathing, a rhythmical form of breathing that can bring harmony into your entire system and is effective in reducing perceived stress.[8] Another suitable breath when dealing with stress is *Ujjayi* Breath (see p.84).

I recommend restorative inversions or hip openers because a lot of people hold stress and tension in their hips. The Sleeping-pigeon Pose, for example, is the perfect antidote to stress and can switch your mind into a more relaxed mode.

All the exercises in this chapter can help to relieve stress, but for more exercises and tips also look at the Anger chapter (see p.15), the Anxiety chapter (see p.29) and the Insomnia chapter (see p.183).

EXERCISES

Cleansing Exercise
(Kriya and Mantra) using sound

This exercise can activate and tone your vagus nerve that is connected to your vocal cords and the muscles at the back of your throat. I love the effect of this *Kundalini Yoga* exercise and practise it whenever I feel stressed.

Caution: Do not practise this exercise if you have a heart condition.

● **Sit down on the floor or on the edge of a chair.** Keep your spine straight and your shoulders relaxed. Bend your arms and tuck your elbows into your ribcage.

● **Make fists with your hands** *(Matsya Mudra),* with your thumbs tucked into your palms. Squeeze your thumbs whenever you produce the sound 'Har', rolling the 'r.' To produce this sound, touch the upper palate of your mouth with the tip of your tongue, so that it can vibrate as you breathe out through your mouth.

● **Next, cross your arms** (left arm on top) and tap your chest with both your fists at the same time, still squeezing the thumbs. Keep on tapping for a maximum of 3 minutes while producing the sound 'Har'.

● **To finish, shake out your arms**, close your eyes and feel the positive relaxing impact of this exercise in your fingers, chest, face and jaw.

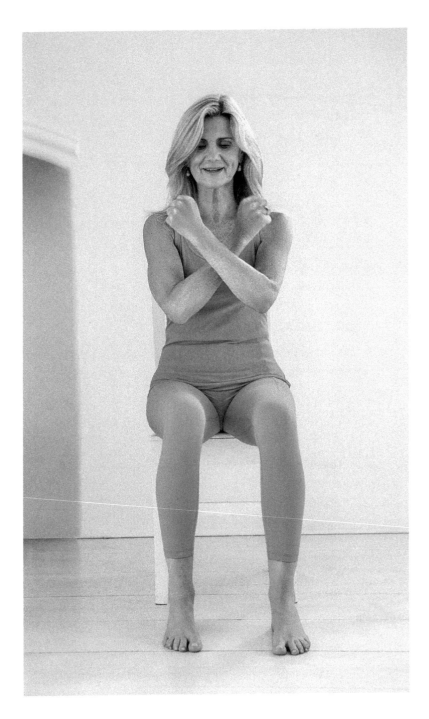

Sleeping-pigeon Pose
(Eka Pada Rajakapotasana)

Enjoy this deeply calming and hip-opening forward bend. Hips are often associated with holding emotional tension and stress, and this posture can help you to let go of both.

Caution: Do not practise this exercise if you have severe problems with your knees or hips.

● **Position yourself on all fours.** Curl your toes under and lift your knees a couple of inches off the floor.

● **Bring your right knee towards your right wrist** and your right foot across and behind your left wrist. Don't worry if your foot is not entirely behind your wrist. Use a yoga block to support your right hip if necessary.

● **Extend your left leg back** and make sure that your hips are square and that your left knee is pointing downwards.

● **Lower your upper body, moving your hands forwards,** in front of your body, which is folding forwards. Create a cushion with your hands and place your forehead onto your hands.

● **Hold the pose for several breaths,** then exit safely: press your hands into the floor and lift your upper body. Tuck your left toes under and come back onto all fours. Repeat on the other side.

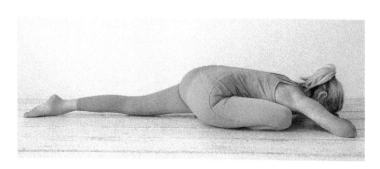

Rhythmic Breath
(Savitri Pranayama)

Holding your breath for just a couple of seconds can help you to get control over your mind and feelings.

Caution: Do not practise this exercise if you are pregnant or suffer from any heart condition, thyroid disorder or respiratory conditions.

- **Sit on a chair or on the floor** with your spine straight. Relax your hands on your thighs and close your eyes, if you want to. Try to breathe in and out through your nose.

- **Start with a ratio of 4:2,** so you breathe in for a count of 4 through your nose, retain your breath for a count of 2, then breathe out for a count of 4 through your nose and hold the breath again for a count of 2.

- **To make this exercise easier, imagine a rectangle.** Move up the left side of the rectangle, breathing in while counting to 4. Turn over to the right side while counting to 2 (holding your breath), moving down the right side for 4 (breathing out) and to the left for 2 (holding the breath).

- **Once you have mastered the ratio of 4:2,** you can change to the emotionally balancing 6:3 or the strengthening ratio of 8:4.

- **Practise this breathing exercise daily** for a couple of minutes.

Corpse Pose (Savasana) and Progressive Muscle Relaxation (PMR)

PMR is a simple and effective technique that can help to reduce stress and muscle tension. It involves tensing and relaxing different muscle groups for 5-10 seconds, before moving onto the next group.

Caution: Be careful if you have muscle or joint problems, cardiovascular conditions or asthma.

- **Lie on the floor** and support your head with a yoga block if necessary. Close your eyes, if you want to, and take a couple of deep and even breaths.

- **Begin by flexing and relaxing your feet.** Squeeze your toes for 5-10 seconds, then release.

- **Move onto your calves and kneecaps**, repeating the process of tensing and relaxing.

- **Continue with your thighs,** glutes, abdomen, back, hands, arms, shoulders and neck - one area after the other.

- **Now, make a surprised expression** with your face. Then, make a grumpy face - squeeze all your facial muscles, sticking out your tongue. Relax your face.

- **Smile for 5-10 seconds.**

- **Repeat this exercise** as often as you like.

FURTHER TIPS

● **Try not to make any assumptions** in moments of stress. Establish the facts.

● **Learn to say NO!** People will eventually understand and respect your boundaries.

● **Work smarter, not harder,** and accept that you will not always have time for everything and everyone.

● **Start making lists.** If you feel easily overwhelmed by your daily workload, sit down and focus on the things that need to be done. Tick off your list at the end of the day and write a new one the next morning.

● **Put a few drops of scented oil on your wrist:** try frankincense, cedar wood, sage, neroli, lemongrass or lavender. All these aromas can help you to de-stress.[9]

● **Consider taking magnesium.** Some people call it 'nature's tranquilliser' because of its ability to induce a relaxing effect within your body.[10]

● **Eat food that is high in omega-3,** including fish, vegetable oils, nuts (especially walnuts), flaxseeds and green leafy vegetables. Omega-3 is necessary for the electrical functioning of your brain and nervous system, and it can increase the activity of the vagus nerve (see p.286).

Avoid multitasking. It just increases stress and nothing gets done properly.

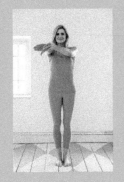

Tennis elbow

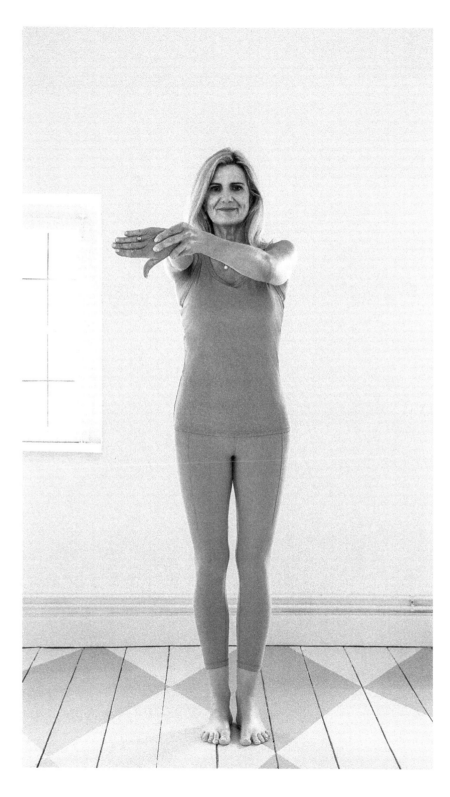

Tennis elbow

"A bad day at tennis is still better than
a good day at work." [1]

(Unknown)

The first time that I experienced tennis elbow was after months of picking up and carrying around my first-born daughter. I only used my left arm to lift her, and she was one chubby baby. Soon a pain started on the outside of my left elbow, and I was unable to do the easiest things anymore, such as brushing my hair or undoing fastenings one-handed. This simple elbow problem meant I had to rely on others to do the most basic things for me and my baby.

Tennis elbow can be surprisingly persistent and last for months, or even years. Even though it is called tennis elbow, only 10% of people affected actually play tennis. The inflammatory condition can be caused by any repetitive motion: painting, chopping ingredients, or using hand tools or a computer mouse. Anyone can get it in both arms, but it usually develops in the one that is used most of the time.

In my case it flared up again and again. I received all kinds of physio. Nothing helped long-term and an operation seemed inevitable. I then decided to take matters into my own hands.

INTRODUCTION

My expectations were low, but with the help of my daily yoga stretches combined with precise cortisone injections, I eventually succeeded in getting rid of my painful condition. At least, so far so good …

My advice: once you notice pain on the outside of your elbow, immediately stop any activities that might aggravate it. Apply ice or a cold pack for 15 minutes 3 times a day.

If you want to continue playing tennis even though you are prone to getting tennis elbow, make sure that you warm up before you start training and use a light racket with a larger grip. Never play with damp or older tennis balls and ice your joints after each game.

Bear in mind that even though yoga can play an important role in managing your tennis elbow, it also can trigger it. Therefore, you need to modify your usual exercises and avoid any weight-bearing poses. So no plank, Upward or Downward-facing Dog Poses. This can narrow your choice of yoga classes and instead of *Ashtanga* flow, I would opt for more static and precise *Iyengar* yoga sessions.

Learn to modify your postures, focusing more on standing extensions such as the Triangle Pose (see p.38) or seated warming up stretches (see Fibromyalgia chapter, p.103).

Some people hope to become more flexible by practising yoga, but do not be fooled by the flexibility of most yogis. A lot of them, me included, are hypermobile. This condition may make us look 'good' in difficult yoga postures, but it also makes us prone to develop problems such as tennis elbow.[2]

EXERCISES

Mountain Pose (Tadasana)

The Mountain Pose serves as the foundational pose for many yoga postures. This time we are using it to focus on stretching your tennis elbow arm. You are going to do the stretches on both arms. You might want to start with the healthy arm.

● **Stand with your feet hip-width apart.** Spread your toes and press your big toes into the floor, lifting your kneecaps and inner thigh muscles. Lengthen your neck, dropping your shoulder blades down towards your tailbone.

● **Extend your right arm out in front of you,** at shoulder height. Flex your wrist with your palm facing towards you and your fingers pointing downwards.

● **Press your left fingers against the top of your right hand,** below your wrist and in line with your right middle finger. Push your right palm towards you with enough pressure for you to feel the stretch. Hold it for 10 deep in- and out-breaths. Relax.

● **For more of a stretch** throughout the entire extended side of your forearm, internally rotate your right shoulder and arm and point all the fingers of your right hand out to the side but without lifting your right shoulder. Again, press against the top of your right hand, below your wrist and in line with your right middle finger (see photo, p296). Hold for 10 breaths.

● **Now, your right arm is down, close to your body.** Flex your right wrist so that your palm is facing up, curving your fingertips up towards the ceiling (as if you secretly receive something). Drop your left ear towards your left shoulder and put your left hand onto your right ear. Hold the stretch for 10 breaths. Repeat all 3 stretches on the other side.

MODIFICATION (HARDER)
You can also perform these stretches positioned on all fours, with your hands directly under your shoulders, your knees under your hips and your head slightly in front of your hands. I prefer to do these stretches using my acupressure mat.

● **Rotate both shoulders and arms inwards,** flex your hands and place your wrists and the top of your hands onto the floor or the acupressure mat. Your fingers are pointing out to the side. Keep your shoulders as squared as possible. Breathe into the stretch and gently move from side to side.

● **To make it easier,** practise just one arm at a time.

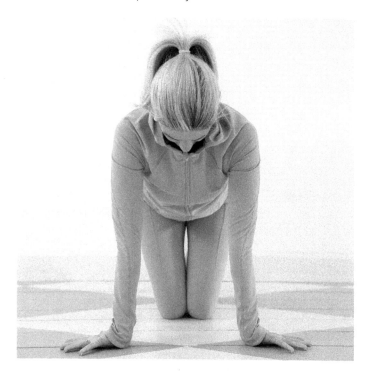

FURTHER TIPS

● **Use an acupressure mat**
to do your arm and wrist
stretches. The needles can
encourage the flow of blood
into your arm and elbow,
therefore supporting the
healing process.[3]

● **Steroid injections** can
provide short-term relief.[4]
However, I suggest that
you mark the exact point
where your pain is located
before the injection. I have
found this most helpful
because the success of the
injection depends on how
precisely the needle gets
to the inflamed point.

● **Consider having PRP
(platelet-rich plasma
injections).** They also
can speed up the healing
process of your tennis
elbow.[5] But it is more costly
than a steroid injection
and might not be offered
straight away.

● **Botox is another option.**
A recent study showed a
consistent and positive
effect of botulinum toxin in
connection with tennis
elbow.[6] Always seek advice
from your GP before having
Botox injections.

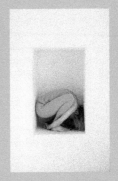

Tinnitus

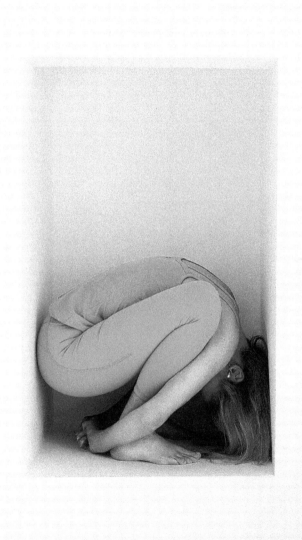

Tinnitus

"I have often lamented that we cannot close our ears with as much ease as which we close our eyes." [1]

Sir Richard Steele (Writer)

One evening I went to bed and woke up in the middle of the night with an annoying buzzing sound inside my ear. First, I tried to ignore it, but the noise was too persistent and after a couple of days I called my GP. He told me to relax and said, 'With a bit of luck it will go away by itself'. It didn't go away, and I was worried that the noise would stay with me forever. The buzzing sound seemed more noticeable because I felt stressed, yet the increasing tinnitus was causing more stress; thus, resulting in a vicious cycle. [2]

The persistent noise comes from the inside, not from an outside source. It is generally believed to originate in the auditory system, which are the ears and parts of the brain responsible for understanding sound.

Tinnitus can affect anybody at any age. Approximately 7.1 million people in the UK live with persistent tinnitus and an estimated 1 million GP consultations take place every year in the UK, with the treatment pathway for tinnitus costing the NHS £750 million. [3]

Can yoga help? Although yoga cannot cure tinnitus once and for all, research indicates that mindfulness and breathing techniques can help to reduce stress and the symptoms of tinnitus.[4] With mindful yoga exercises, you can create some space from the ringing noise, and in that space you can decide how you are going to respond to the sound in your ear.

In my case, I practised the exercises in this chapter daily and, after a couple of months, my perception of the noise started to change - the whooshing and buzzing faded and eventually stopped. There is no guarantee, but it is worth trying.

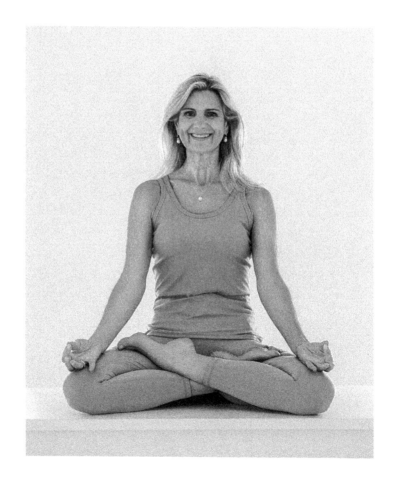

EXERCISES

Relax with Mindfulness

Listen to the noise in your ear. Have you ever just observed it without discrimination, emotional judgement or thought? Probably not. Therefore, take a moment and try to neutrally observe the noise, not identifying with it, simply just noting it.

● **Sit comfortably,** preferably on the edge of a chair, with your spine straight, your feet touching the floor, your shoulders relaxed and your eyes closed.

● **Slowly, shift your awareness** away from the noise in your ear to your audible breath. You can use *Ujjayi*, the Ocean Sound Breath (see p.84), or simply focus on an even in- and out-breath through both nostrils. Concentrate solely on your breath and if your mind drifts away to the noise in your ear, acknowledge that, and then guide your focus back to your breathing.

● **The going back to your breath** can happen once or hundreds of times. The breath is always there; the noise is only there when observed. The more space you make between yourself and the noise in your ear, the less attached to the noise you will be, and the more you will be able to focus your awareness on other sensations.

● **Practise this mindful relaxation** every day for the next 3 months for a couple of minutes.

Ear Pressing and Tapping

Tapping (see p.40) can unblock the flow of energy within your body and it is a yogic belief that when the energy, *Prana*, flows freely, your body and mind will be able to heal itself.

Tapping acupressure points with your fingertips can reduce the stimulation of the limbic system in your brain that deals with emotions, memories and behaviours, particularly the survival behaviours. The limbic system can act as a gatekeeper to keep the tinnitus signal from reaching the auditory cortex, which is the part of your brain responsible for your perception of sounds.[5]

● **Sit comfortably with your spine straight.** Press your right thumb against your tragus, the small cartilage in front of your ear canal. Push your thumb against it, approximately 50 times in quick succession.

● **Stop pushing** and now press your thumb firmly against the small cartilage. Hold it, slowly counting to 12, then release.

● **Now, do the same** with your left thumb on your left ear, before repeating the techniques on both ears simultaneously.

● **Then, tuck in your chin** and use your fingertips, not your fingernails, to tap firmly against your skull behind your ears. Relax your jaw muscles and lips while tapping forcefully for at least 30 seconds.

● **Move your fingertips to the crown of your head** and tap the top of your head for a further 30 seconds.

● **To finish, tap your chin for 30 seconds** before repeating the whole ritual.

● **Practise twice a day** for a couple of months until you notice an improvement.

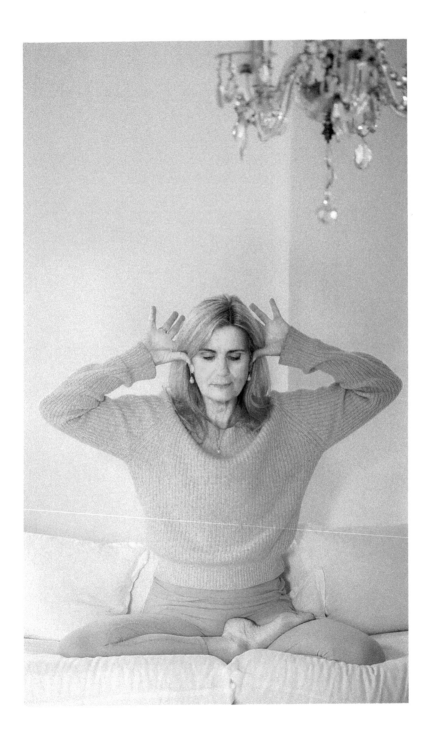

Humming Bee Breath (Bhramari)

This technique involves making a humming sound while breathing. The vibrations and sound you make can distract you from the ringing and buzzing sound in your ears.

Caution: Do not practise this exercise if you suffer from migraines or any heart ailment.

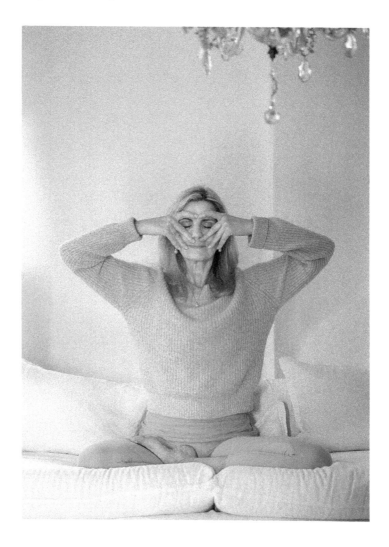

- **Keep your jaw relaxed,** with your lips gently closed and your teeth slightly apart throughout this exercise.

- **If it feels comfortable, close your eyes.** Push your thumbs against your tragus, the cartilage in front of your ear canal. Place your index fingers above each eyebrow. Bring your middle fingers beside each nostril, but do not block your nose. Relax your ring fingers next to your mouth.

- **Keep your ears and lips softly closed** and produce a humming sound as you breathe out. Produce the sound 'm' and sustain the sound until you need to inhale again.

- **Continue to inhale through your nose** and hum like a buzzing bee as you exhale: 'mmmmmmm …' Do not clench your teeth and do not press the tongue against your teeth as you are humming.

- **Listen to the sound and notice** the tingling on your lips, face and skull. The longer you can maintain the humming bee exhalation, the more relaxing the breath is likely to be. Listen to the humming sound for at a couple of minutes.

- **To finish, release your hands,** extend your legs and spend a few moments breathing normally. Sit quietly and notice whether there are any changes to the sound in your ears.

Cobra Pose
(Bhujangasana)

In this posture the lengthening of your neck can help to open your ear canal, which in turn can alleviate the ringing noise in your ear.

Caution: Do not practise this exercise if you are pregnant, or if you have severe back problems.

● **Lie on your front** with your hands flat on the floor underneath your shoulders. Exhale and slowly raise your head, shoulders and upper chest off the floor, without using your hands.

● **As you lift, squeeze your buttock muscles.** Press your pubic bone into the floor to prevent compressing your lower back.

● **Try to keep the back of your head in line with your spine,** lengthening your neck and spine.

● **Once you have found the correct height,** take your hands off the floor, and tuck your elbows in. Hold the pose for approximately 10 in-breaths and 10 out-breaths.

● **To finish,** lie flat on your tummy, turn your head to the right side and then the left side, before pushing yourself up into Child's Pose (see p.241).

FURTHER TIPS

● **Take sufficient Vitamin B12** and Ginkgo Biloba. These supplements can help with tinnitus.[6, 7]

● **Avoid consuming caffeine,** nicotine and alcohol, as they can all increase your blood pressure, which can make the ringing more evident.

● **Go to bed and listen to calming music,** enabling you to fall asleep more easily.

● **Consider having Cognitive Behavioural Therapy (**CBT). It might not influence the symptoms of tinnitus, but it can help to improve your response to it.[8]

● **Talk to others** and find a support group. For more information, consult Tinnitus UK. Tel: 0114 250 9933. https://tinnitus.org.uk

The more space you make between yourself and the noise in your ear, the less attached to the noise you will be.

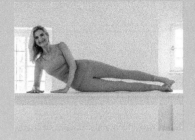

Weight loss

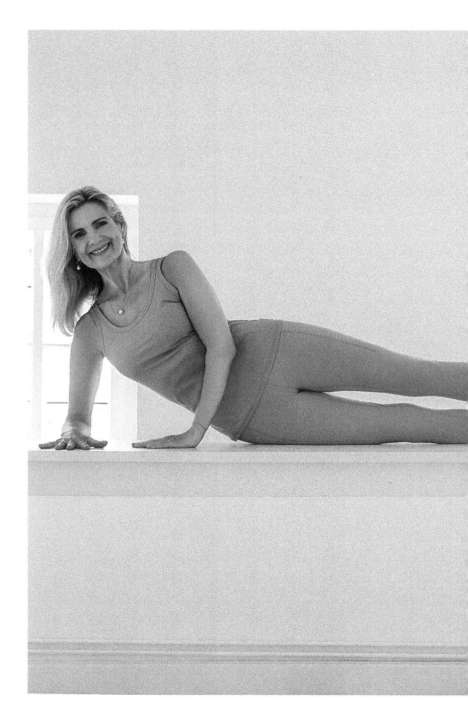

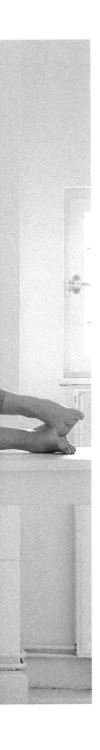

Weight loss

"You have to make the decision to lose weight in your head, not your stomach." [1]

Jean Nidetch (Entrepreneur)

I have always been slim, which is nothing to be proud of, as it is just part of my genetic make-up. However, recently I have put on some weight, especially around my hips and waist. Does it bother me? Yes. I am not keen on having belly rolls, and it slightly annoys me that I do not fit into my favourite jeans anymore. Do I want to change? No. Even though I would like to lose a couple of kilos, I am not prepared to cut down on food and drinks. However, I am willing to exercise a bit more than usual, so I can strengthen and tone my body to feel more dynamic again.

Before you decide to lose weight, ask yourself why. It should not be because you want to fulfil anybody's expectations, but because you want to feel better and live longer. If that is the case, then start losing weight now.

It might come as a surprise, but the UK is one of the 'fattest' nations in Europe! [2] There has been a lot of press recently about how our diet is particularly high in Ultra Processed Foods (UPF), which certainly needs to be considered as part of the problem. Almost three-quarters of people aged 45-74 are overweight or obese. Being heavy can shorten your life expectancy, as it is associated with cardiovascular disease and cancer. Furthermore, too much weight can be connected to type 2 diabetes, hypertension, sleep apnoea, reflux, arthritis, polycystic ovary syndrome and infertility.[3] So, is there a silver lining? Yes, a regular yoga practice can help you to maintain or lose weight. But bear in mind that the yogic approach and process of weight loss is rather slow and requires discipline and patience.

The best yoga practice to lose weight is a whole sequence of different postures, which can work your heart and every muscle in your body, increasing your metabolism and reducing levels of cortisol. This is relevant because elevated cortisol levels can lead to an increase in appetite and weight. Furthermore, flowing movements like the Sun Salutation can stimulate the production of irisin, a hormone that seems to help weight loss.[4, 5]

However, all the exercise in the world cannot make up for taking on more calories than you burn. So, consider a fresh approach to your eating habits; forget past diets and frustration, and discover moderation and enjoyment of food. This more yogic approach can help you to accelerate weight loss – not quickly, but efficiently and long-term.

Plan what you want to eat and look forward to it! The worst thing that can happen is that you get so hungry that you literally stuff your face with whatever food you can get quickly. Admittedly that can be me, after a day of work without a lunch break. Whether alone or in company, eat with awareness, consciously taking your time. Try not to feel guilty and learn to appreciate each bite. This so-called 'mindful eating' can help you to become more aware of your feelings and the physical sensations related to eating. In addition, combine mindful eating with a concept called intermittent fasting (IF) – 16:8 fasting is generally considered safe, but talk to your GP before giving it a go, especially if you have any underlying health issues. Be careful with diabetes, low blood pressure or low blood-sugar levels, and do not restrict your food intake at all if you are pregnant. This way of eating allows you to eat whatever you like within an 8-hour window. It can help you to lose weight and reduce the risk of leptin (a hunger hormone) resistance, which can be a key risk factor for obesity. Between meals, if you don't snack, your insulin levels will go down and your fat cells can then release their stored sugar, to be used as energy. The entire idea of IF is to allow the insulin levels to go down far enough and for long enough so that you can burn off fat.[6, 7]

Of course, it is still important to eat and live as healthily as possible during the allowed time frame! This means lots of fresh vegetables, fruit and sensible portions of protein to keep you fuller for longer, as 16 hours of fasting won't compensate for 8 hours of stuffing your face with sugary processed junk food and no additional exercise.[8]

If in doubt about what kind of food is best for you, side with the Ayurvedic perspective, which believes that everyone has a different constitution and it can be most helpful to learn whether you are a *Kapha*, *Pitta* or *Vata* type (see p.330). *Kapha*-dominated people, for example, can struggle with their weight more than the often-fiery *Pitta* or the nervous *Vata* types. Once you have determined your *Doshic* type, you will be able to find the most suitable way of practising yoga and you will find out which food brings out the best in you.[9]

Breathing techniques can be an effective weight loss tool. Bellows Breath, *Bhastrika*, a full rapid breathing technique. can raise your metabolism (meaning you burn fat faster) and can correct any imbalances in your 3 *Doshas*. If you do this regularly over 8 weeks, research has shown that you can reduce your waist–hip ratio and body mass index (BMI).[10]

EXERCISES

Bellows Breath
(Bhastrika)

Ideally practise this revitalising breathing exercise early in the morning to set yourself up for a successful day. The Bellows Breath is a powerful yoga tool. It is better to do fewer repetitions with equal vigour than too many repetitions because your breath will become weaker and less effective.

Caution: Do not practise *Bhastrika* if you are pregnant or if you have untreated high blood pressure, any heart issues, a hernia or ulcers. People with asthma or chronic bronchitis need to be careful.

- **Blow your nose** before you start the exercise.

- **Sit comfortably on the floor** or on the edge of a chair with your feet below your knees, in a stable position with your back and neck straight.

- **Ensure that nothing is restricting your belly.** Relax your hands in a diamond shape on your lower abdomen, with your thumbs pointing towards your navel.

- **Breathe in through your nose** and notice how your belly fully expands. Breathe out through your nose and feel a gentle contraction as your belly moves towards your spine. Focus on both the inhalation and exhalation equally. Repeat 5 more times.

WEIGHT LOSS

Bhastrika, a full rapid breathing technique, can raise your metabolism, helping you to burn fat faster.

● **Now, breathe in and out faster,** more forcefully. Breathe in energetically and breathe out vigorously through both nostrils.

● **As you breathe in,** feel your belly pushing against your hands. As you breathe out, feel the tightening of your abdominal muscles. Try to keep your mouth shut throughout the exercise, with just your belly, nostrils and the little notch in your throat moving, but not your shoulders.

● **Practise up to 10 breaths,** gradually increasing to 25 repetitions daily.

Sun Salutation (Surya Namaskar)

I recommend starting your daily exercise routine with 3 sets of the Sun Salutation, gradually building up to 6, 9 and eventually 12. A set of exercises consists of 2 rounds: the first round you start and finish with the right leg, the second round you start and finish with the left leg. Start slowly to warm up your body and focus on taking even in- and out-breaths in harmony with your movement.

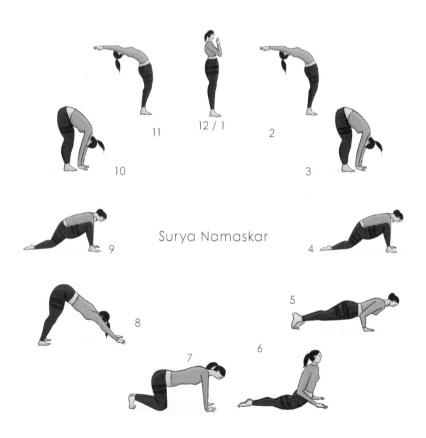

Surya Namaskar

1 Breathe in and out in Mountain Pose (*Tadasana*) (see p.78).

2 Breathe in for Standing Backward Bend (see photo, p.168).

3 Breathe out as you swan-dive into Standing Forward Bend (*Uttanasana*) (see p.188).

4 Breathe in as you step into Runner's Lunge Pose (*Anjaneyasana*).

5 Breathe out, step back the other leg into Plank Pose (*Chaturanga Dandasana*). Hold the Plank Pose for a couple of breaths.

6 Breathe out, drop your knees, lower your chest, then move up into Cobra Pose (*Bhujangasana*) (see p.312), breathing in.

7 Breathe out as you push up onto all fours, into Tabletop Lift (*Bharmanasana*) (see p.97).

8 Breathe in and lift your knees. Breathe out, hold the Tabletop Pose and breathe in as you come into Downward-facing Dog (*Adho Mukha Svanasana*) (see p.151). Hold the pose for a couple of breaths, if you like, then drop your knees and come onto all fours.

9 Breathe in, step forward with your right leg into Runner's Lunge Pose.

10 Breathe out and step forward with your left leg into Standing Forward Bend Pose.

11 Breathe in and roll up into Standing Backward Bend Pose.

12 Breathe out and finish in the Mountain Pose.

Repeat the 12 poses, starting with your left leg. Finish standing with your hands folded in front of your chest, *Namaste*. This completes one round of the Sun Salutation.

Food Meditation

It is hard to believe but, according to a recent study, listening to your food can help you lose weight.[11] Try it with your favourite food, the crunchier the better.

● **Prepare your food on a plate,** appreciating the energy that went into its production. Now, sit in front of it. Look at your food – its texture and colour. Then, close your eyes and smell the food until your mouth starts watering. Swallow your saliva, open your mouth and begin to eat, listening and chewing each bite for at least 20 seconds.

● **Pause for a moment,** before you continue eating.

● **Repeat the chewing and listening** as often as you like.

● **If listening to food does not appeal to you,** then simply chew your food, while counting slowly to 20 before you swallow.

● **Occasionally remind yourself** that food is not an enemy but your trusted friend. A friend you choose wisely. And how you eat is just as important as what and when you eat.[12] (See Fat Belly chapter, p.87 and Reflux chapter, p.253.)

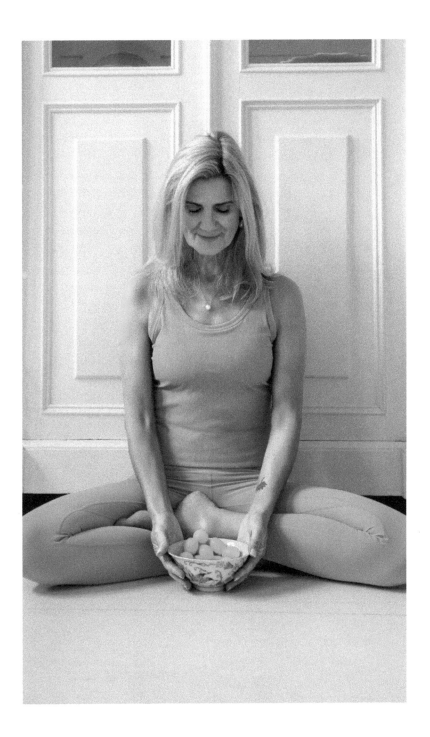

FURTHER TIPS

● **Keep a food diary,** which could act as a form of self-study, called *Svadhyaya*. You might notice that just by writing down your food consumption every day that you will eat less.

● **Cut out crisps** for a while. No other nation in Europe is so obsessed from an early age with the consumption of crisps. You will never lose weight if you continue to eat crisps. One pack of crisps a day is the equivalent of drinking 5 litres (8.799 pints) of cooking oil per year. Nearly a fifth of British children eat 2 packets of crisps a day and that might explain the soaring rates of obesity among children.[13]

● **Drink lots of still water** and unsweetened herbal tea during the day and before mealtimes.

● **Cut out sugar!** It can have a dramatic and positive effect on your weight and cravings.[14]

● **Sleep a lot.** And if you wake up in the middle of the night, opt for sex rather than food. Even the most relaxing missionary position can burn up to 100 calories, and when you go on top you will burn even more, up to 150 calories.

● **Look into dietary supplements** such as choline and inositol. A research study found that choline can play an important role in the metabolism of fat, encouraging body mass reduction.[15] Furthermore, ask your GP about metformin. This wasn't designed to be a weight loss drug, but researchers have found a link between metformin and weight loss. Studies concluded that the safe diabetes drug could serve as a treatment for excess body weight.[16]

Enjoy yoga, move
your body and
nourish your soul to
empower your health
and wellbeing.

APPENDIX

CHAKRAS

You cannot see, smell, hear or taste it, but everyone is full of it: *Prana*, our life force. The energy travels through our bodies via thousands of channels, called *Nadis*. What the veins may be for blood, the *Nadis* are for *Prana*. These *Nadis* culminate and come together in *Chakras*, energy centres. You can imagine chakras like spinning discs that should stay open and move in harmony with each other for your optimal physical and emotional wellbeing. If chakras become blocked, it can trigger physical, mental or emotional imbalance. Yoga exercises, breathing and meditation all can help to clear *Nadis* for *Prana* to move through them freely. And a free flow of energy can then re-establish an equilibrium that may support you in your wellbeing.[1] There is no scientific proof about chakras and their impact on our health, but some studies suggest that the chakra system can be a vital key for modern psychology, neuropsychology and healing.[2]

To restore balance within your chakras, first tune in to how you are feeling. Then, figure out which chakra to stimulate to counteract any imbalance. For example, if you are feeling low in energy, you can do poses that stimulate your navel chakra to reignite your inner fire. But if you are feeling anxious and need to feel more grounded, you can choose poses for the earthy Root Chakra. Or if you seek more courage and confidence, you can opt for poses that open and stimulate your Throat Chakra.

Here is a general overview of the 7 main chakras and their potential impact on organs and body parts according to yogic beliefs. Starting from the base of your spine:

- *Sahasrara* (Crown Chakra)
- *Ajna* (Third-Eye Chakra)
- *Vishuddha* (Throat Chakra)
- *Anahata* (Heart Chakra)
- *Manipura* (Solar Plexus Chakra)
- *Swadhisthana* (Sacral Chakra)
- *Muladhara* (Root Chakra)

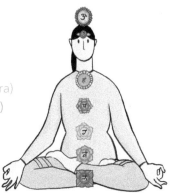

Sahasrara Chakra, located at the top of your head. Yogis believe that this is your entrance to the divine. This energy centre can correspond with your pineal gland and nervous system. Its element is pure consciousness.

Ajna Chakra, located between your eyebrows. This is the so-called third eye, seat of intuition and clarity of thought. It can affect your pituitary gland, brain, vision, ears and nose. Its element is light.

Vishuddha Chakra, located in your throat and neck. This is the seat of communication and self-expression. Your vocal cords, neck and thyroid can be affected by this chakra. Its element is ether, or space.

Anahata Chakra, located right at the centre of your chest. This is the seat of devotion and love. Your heart, thymus gland, lungs and your circulatory system can be influenced by this energy centre. Its element is air.

Manipura Chakra, located in the upper abdomen, around your navel. This is the seat of your power, control and confidence. The stomach, pancreas, liver, gall bladder and small intestine can be affected by this energy centre. Its element is fire.

Swadhisthana Chakra, located in your lower abdomen, below your navel, is the seat of your emotions, sexual energy and creativity. Your reproductive organs, bladder and your lower back can be affected by this chakra. Its element is water.

Muladhara Chakra, located at the base of your spine. Your bones, muscles, teeth, skin, kidneys, adrenal glands, large intestine, legs and feet can be affected by this energy centre. This chakra refers to your survival instincts, sense of security and stability. Its element is the earth.

AYURVEDA DOSHA TEST

I have based this test on the *Ayurveda Dosha* Test from the *Ayurveda Encyclopedia*.[3] *Ayurveda* is the Indian science of self-healing and it has evolved alongside yoga over thousands of years. Vital to *Ayurveda* is the concept of *Dosha*, an individual's mental and physical constitution. There are 3 types of *Doshas*, known as *Vata* (air/ether), *Pitta* (fire/water) and *Kapha* (earth/water). To maintain a balanced ratio of all 3 *Doshas* is considered one of the best ways to stay healthy and happy (see p.256).

Usually, one of the *Doshas* will dominate over the others. To determine your *Doshic* type, simply count how many ticks you get for each *Dosha* in the chart opposite. The *Dosha* with the most ticks predominates. If 2 or 3 suggestions in a category apply equally, tick them all. If none applies, tick none. At the end, count all your points.

Once you know your *Doshic* type, you can adjust your lifestyle, diet and yoga practice to get the best out of your constitution and to feel more balanced and stronger.

If *Vata* is dominating your life, try not to exercise too vigorously. Rather feel centred in standing poses and work from your midline with steadiness and ease. Your breath should remain

	VATA	PITTA	KAPHA
BODY FRAME	thin, medium	medium	medium, large
WEIGHT	light, bony	medium, muscular	medium, heavy
SKIN	dry, thin	warm, freckles	pale, moist
FACE SHAPE	long, oval	heart shape	round or square
EYES	rather small	piercing	large
LIPS	thin, dry	soft, pink	large, smooth
NOSE	thin, long	sharp, pointed	straight, thick
TONGUE	rough	red, dark	white
HAIR	dry, thin	oily, thin	thick, wavy
NAILS	rough, brittle	soft, pink	soft, white
TEETH	uneven	medium, yellow	large, even
JOINTS	stiff	flexible	strong
SWEATING	little	a lot	moderate
STOOL	small, hard	loose	solid
APPETITE	variable	strong	constant, low
PULSE	80-100	70-80	60-70
MEMORY	poor long-term	good, sharp	good long-term
SPEECH	quick, talkative	clear, abrupt	slow, silent
SLEEP	light	moderate	deep
LIFESTYLE	erratic	busy	steady
BELIEFS	radical	leader	loyal
ENDURANCE	poor	moderate	excellent
SEXUALITY	can be cold	intense	warm, constant
TEMPERAMENT	nervous	impatient	easy going
EMOTIONS	enthusiastic, worries	warm, can get angry	calm, attached
FINANCES	spends on trifles	spends on luxury	saves money
POINTS			

slow and even throughout your movements. Furthermore, eat lots of warm and nourishing food, such as cooked vegetables, nuts, rice, oats, beans and tofu. Avoid dried fruits, apples, hard cheese, frozen vegetables, white sugar, chocolate and anything gas-forming.

If *Pitta* seems to rule your life, then try not to be over-competitive in your yoga practice. Instead, fiery *Pittas* can benefit from a calming, restorative yoga practice, with emphasis on inversions and twisting poses.

Excess *Pitta* is best balanced by a diet of fresh whole foods, cooked and raw, that is cooling and hearty. Eat more soft cheese, ice cream, yoghurt, green vegetables, cereals, beans and pulses. Avoid grapefruit, salted butter, hard cheese, sour cream, horseradish, garlic, peppers, nuts and anything too spicy.

Kapha people need to keep moving. Preferably they should break into a little sweat while doing yoga exercises. Focus on standing postures, practise yoga sequences like the Sun Salutation (see p.322) and minimise seated positions. Use a rapid breath to maintain energy and to increase your metabolism. Too much *Kapha* is best adjusted by consuming a diet of freshly cooked whole foods that are light, dry, warming, well spiced and relatively easy to digest.

Try to eat more apples and pears, low-fat soft cheese, sunflower seeds, popcorn, barley, rye and honey. Avoid banana, kiwi, watermelon, squash, pumpkin, tomatoes, cucumber, butter, ice cream, full-fat yoghurt, avocado, wheat, oats, and anything mucus-forming.[4]

PROPS

The props you need can vary, depending on the style of yoga and the level of your practice. Some props simply enhance your exercise and provide comfort and support.

- **A non-slip yoga mat,** which you can wash regularly in the washing machine.

- **2 yoga bricks.** I prefer the cork to the foam ones because they feel safer and sturdier.

- **1 yoga block.**

- **A yoga strap** can assist you in stretching. An extra-long one with a metallic instead of a plastic buckle is easier to adjust.

- **A yoga bolster** is a beautiful device to have, not just for restorative yoga poses.

- **A spiky acupressure mat** is my favourite tool, but better to try one first, before you buy one.

- **Two 1kg weights.**

- **A silk eye pillow.**

- **A blanket.**

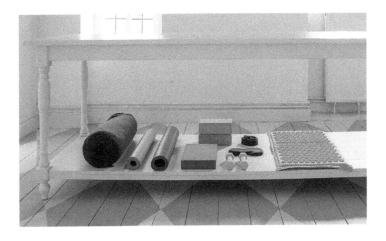

REFERENCES

THE BEGINNING

1 Theodor W. Adorno (1903–1969) was a German philosopher, sociologist, psychologist and composer. Quote sourced from buboquote.com.

ANGER

1 Vladimiro Ariel Dorfman (born 1942) is an Argentine Chilean American novelist, playwright, essayist, academic and human rights activist. Quote sourced from BrainyQuote.com.

2 Staicu ML, Cuțov M. 'Anger and health risk behaviours'. J Med Life. 2010 Oct–Dec;3(4):372-5. PMID: 21254733; PMCID: PMC3019061.

3 Chapman BP, et al. 'Emotion suppression and mortality risk over a 12-year follow-up'. J Psychosom Res. 2013; 75(4): 381-385. Doi: 10.1016/j.jpsychores.2013.07.014.

4 Propper RE, et al (2013) 'Getting a Grip on Memory: Unilateral Hand Clenching Alters Episodic Recall'. PLOS ONE 8(5): 10.1371/annotation/693ff849 -c230-4e59-8772-b8755daf0f75.

5 Muktibodhananda, S. Hatha Yoga Pradipika, chapter two, Bihar School of Yoga, India, 1993.

6 Saraswati, SS. Asana, Pranayama, Mudra Bandha, Yoga Publications Trust, Munger, Bihar, India, 1996. Forward bending asanas, p.227.

7 Strean WB. 'Laughter prescription'. Can Fam Physician. 2009 Oct; 55(10): 965-7. PMID: 19826144; PMCID: PMC2762283.

8 Ruiz DM. The four Agreements: A practical guide to personal freedom. Amber-Allen Publishing. Inc, San Rafael, California, 1997.

9 Janov A. The Primal Scream, Kessinger Publishing, LLC 2007.

ANXIETY

1 P. Murali Doraiswamy (born 1963), Professor of Psychiatry and Behavioural Sciences, is a leading physician scientist in mental health, cognitive neuroscience and mind-body medicine. In an email from September 2020, he kindly allowed me to quote him.

2 Arias-de la Torre J, et al. 'Prevalence and variability of current depressive disorder in 27 European countries: a population-based study'. The Lancet 2021; 6: e729-38, May 4, 2021 https://doi.org/10.1016/S2468-2667(21)00047-5'

3 The Lancet. 'Global prevalence and burden of depressive and anxiety disorders in 204 countries and territories in 2020 due to the COVID-19 pandemic'. Published Online October 8, 2021 https://doi.org/10.1016/ S0140-6736(21)02143-7.

4 Rew, K. 'Risks of Cold Water – Cold shock, cold incapacitation and hypothermia: a beginner's guide to cold risk'. https://www.outdoorswimmingsociety.com/risks-cold-water/

5 Van Tulleken C, et al. 'Open water swimming as a treatment for major depressive disorder'. BMJ Case Rep. 2018;2018:bcr2018225007. Published 2018 Aug 21. doi:10.1136/bcr-2018-225007.

6 Breit S, et al. 'Vagus Nerve as Modulator of the Brain-Gut Axis in Psychiatric and Inflammatory Disorders. Front Psychiatry'. 2018;9:44. Published 2018 Mar 13. doi:10.3389/fpsyt.2018.00044.

7 Gerritsen RJS, Band GPH. 'Breath of Life: The Respiratory Vagal Stimulation Model of Contemplative Activity'. Front Hum Neurosci. 2018 Oct 9; 12:397. doi: 10.3389/fnhum.2018.00397. PMID: 30356789; PMCID: PMC6189422.

8 Smith C, et al. 'A randomised comparative trial of yoga and relaxation to reduce stress and anxiety'. Complement Ther Med. 2007 Jun;15(2):77-83. doi: 10.1016/j.ctim.2006.05.001. Epub 2006 Jun 21. PMID: 17544857.

9 Gibbons, K. 'Battling anxiety? Calls for doctors to prescribe it on the NHS.Yoga is just as effective as a therapy session, say experts'. *The Times*, August 12, 2020.

10 Yackle K, et al. 'Breathing control centre neurons that promote arousal in mice'. *Science*. 2017; 355(6332): 1411-1415. Doi: 10.1126/science.aai7984.

11 Patanjali. *The Yoga Sutras of Patanjali*. Integral Yoga Publications, 1978.

12 Bach D, et al. 'Clinical EFT (Emotional Freedom Techniques) Improves Multiple Physiological Markers of Health'. *J Evid Based Integral Med*. 2019; 24:2515690X18823691. doi:10.1177/2515690X18823691.

13 Keng SL, et al. 'Effects of mindfulness on psychological health: a review of empirical studies'. *Clin Psychol Rev*. 2011 Aug;31(6):1041-56. doi: 10.1016/j.cpr.2011.04.006. Epub 2011 May 13. PMID: 21802619; PMCID: PMC3679190.

14 Guyon AJAA, et al. 'Respiratory Variability, Sighing, Anxiety, and Breathing Symptoms in Low- and High-Anxious Music Students Before and After Performing'. *Front Psychol*. 2020;11:303. Published 2020 Feb 26. doi:10.3389/fpsyg.2020.00303.

15 Koulivand PH, et al. 'Lavender and the nervous system'. *Evid Based Complement Alternat Med*. 2013;2013:681304 doi:10.1155/2013/681304.

16 Krishnakumar D, et al. 'Meditation and Yoga can Modulate Brain Mechanisms that affect Behavior and Anxiety: A Modern Scientific Perspective'. *Anc Sci*. 2015 Apr;2(1):13-19. doi: 10.14259/as. v2i1.171. PMID: 26929928; PMCID: PMC4769029.

17 Fernando Marmolejo-Ramos F. et al. 'Facial Action Influences the Perception of Emotional Faces and Biological Motion Stimuli'. *Experimental Psychology* (2020), 67, pp.14-22.

18 Berceli D, et al. 'Effects of Self-induced Unclassified Therapeutic Tremors on Quality of Life Among Non-professional Caregivers: A Pilot Study. *Glob Adv Health Med*. 2014;3(5):45-48. doi:10.7453/gahmj.2014.032.

19 MacMillan A, Brickell S. 'Weighted Blanket Use: A Systematic Review'. *Am J Occup Ther.*, 2020 Mar/Apr; 74(2):7402205010p1-740220 5010p14. doi: 10.5014/ajot.2020. 037358.

20 Nuss P. 'Anxiety disorders and GABA neurotransmission: a disturbance of modulation'. *Neuropsychiatr Dis Treat*. 2015 Jan 17; 11:165-75. doi: 10.2147/NDT.S58841. PMID: 25653526; PMCID: PMC4303399.

21 Fuladi S, et al. 'Assessment of the Efficacy of Withania somniferous Root Extract in Patients with Generalized Anxiety Disorder: A Randomized Double-blind Placebo-Controlled Trial'. *Curr Rev Clin Exp Pharmacol*. 2021;16(2):191-196. doi: 10.2174/1574884715666200413120413. PMID: 32282308.

22 Mukai T, et al. 'A meta-analysis of inositol for depression and anxiety disorders'. *Psychopharmacology* 2014; 29(1): 55-63.

BACK PAIN

1 Marni Jackson (born 1947) is a Canadian journalist and broadcaster. She is the author of the bestselling book *Pain. The Fifth Vital Sign: The Science and Culture of Why We Hurt,* Random House, 2003. Quote sourced from '7 Quotes from Experts That Will Change How You Look at Back Pain'.

2 Rubin DI. 'Epidemiology and risk factors for spine pain'. *Neurol Clin*. 2007 May; 25(2): 353-71. doi: 10.1016/j.ncl.2007.01.004. PMID: 17445733.

3 Chang DG, et al. 'Yoga as a treatment for chronic low back pain: A systematic review of the literature'. *J Orthop Rheumatol.* 2016 Jan 1;3(1):1-8. PMID: 27231715; PMCID: PMC4878447.

4 NHS. 'Alexander technique'. https://www.nhs.uk/conditions/alexander-technique/

5 Hohmann C, et al. 'The benefit of a mechanical needle stimulation pad in patients with chronic neck and lower back pain: two randomized controlled pilot studies'. *Evid Based Complement Alternat Med.* 2012; 2012:753583. doi: 10.1155/2012/753583. Epub 2012 Sep 11. PMID: 22997531; PMCID: PMC3446809.

6 Little P, et al. 'Randomised controlled trial of Alexander technique lessons, exercise, and massage (ATEAM) for chronic and recurrent back pain'. *BMJ* 2008; 337: a884.

7 Hanscom D. *Back in control. A surgeon's roadmap out of chronic pain,* Vertus Press, Seattle, 2017.

8 Chung MK, Campbell JN. 'Use of Capsaicin to Treat Pain: Mechanistic and Therapeutic Considerations'. *Pharmaceuticals (Basel).* 2016;9(4):66. Published 2016 Nov 1. doi:10.3390/ph9040066.

CONSTIPATION

1 Marvin Gaye was an American singer (1939–1984), songwriter and record producer. He helped to shape the sound of Motown in the 1960s. Quote sourced from Goodreads.com.

2 Forootan M, et al. 'Chronic constipation: A review of literature'. *Medicine,* (Baltimore). 2018; 97(20): e10631. doi:10.1097/MD.000000 0000010631.

3 Bharucha AE, et al. 'American gastroenterological association technical review on constipation'. *Gastroenterology,* 2013; 144:218–38.

4 Bhattacharya S, Chattu VK, Singh A. Health promotion and prevention of bowel disorders through toilet designs: A myth or reality? J Educ Health Promot. 2019;8:40. Published 2019 Feb 15. doi:10.4103/jehp. jehp_198_18

5 Turan, N. 'The Effect of Abdominal Massage on Constipation and Quality of Life'. *Gasteroenterol Nurs.,* 2016 Jan-Feb;39(1):48-59. doi: 10.1097/SGA.00000000 00000202.

6 Badgujar SB, et al. 'Foeniculum vulgare Mill: a review of its botany, phytochemistry, pharmacology, contemporary application, and toxicology'. *Biomed Res Int.* 2014; 2014:842674. doi: 10.1155/2014/842674.

EATING DISORDERS

1 Andrew "Freddie" Flintoff MBE (born 1977). The Ashes-winning cricket hero said he hadn't been in control of his eating for 20 years. Quote sourced from *Radio Times* 'Freddie Flintoff praised for incredibly courageous bulimia documentary" on BBC One'. Flintoff talks about his battle with the eating disorder that primarily involves binge-eating and forced vomiting, but can also manifest itself with abuse of laxatives and excessive exercise routines.

2 Arcelus J, et al. 'Mortality rates in patients with anorexia nervosa and other eating disorders. A meta-analysis of 36 studies'. *Arch Gen Psychiatry,* 2011 Jul;68(7):724-31. doi: 10.1001/archgenpsychiatry. 2011.74. PMID: 21727255.

3 Beat Eating Disorders, beateatingdisorders.org.uk.

4 Karlsen, KE et al. 'Effect of Yoga in the Treatment of Eating Disorders: A Single-blinded Randomized Controlled Trial with 6-Months Follow-up'. *International Journal of Yoga,* vol. 11,2 (2018): 166-169. doi:10.4103/ijoy.IJOY_3_17.

5 Hoffman ER, et al. 'Reproductive issues in anorexia nervosa'. *Expert Rev Obstet Gynecol.,* 2011;6(4): 403-414. doi:10.1586/eog.11.31.

6 Bulik CM, et al. 'Fertility and reproduction in women with anorexia nervosa: a controlled study'. *J Clin Psychiatry*, 1999 Feb;60(2):130-5; quiz 135-7. doi: 10.4088/jcp.v60n0212. PMID: 10084645.

7 Kim YR, et al. 'The impact of intranasal oxytocin on attention to social emotional stimuli in patients with anorexia nervosa: a double blind within-subject cross-over experiment.' *PLoS One*, 2014;9(6):e90721, 2014, Mar 6. doi:10.1371/journal.pone.0090721.

8 Lichtenfeld, S, et al. 'Fertile Green: Green Facilitates Creative Performance'. *Personality and Social Psychology Bulletin*, 2012, vol. 38, no. 6, pp. 784-797.

9 Kass AE, et al. 'Psychological treatments for eating disorders'. *Curr Opin Psychiatry*, 2013;26(6):549-555. doi:10.1097/YCO.0b013e328365a30e.

FAT BELLY

1 Daisy Lowe (born 1989) is an English fashion model and the daughter of songwriter Pearl Lowe and musician Gavin Rossdale. Quote sourced from Starsquotes.com 'Daisy Lowe Quotes About Life, Love, Fabulous, Mabuse, Ability'.

2 Harvard Health Publishing. 'Abdominal obesity and your health'. January 20, 2017.

3 Chen, G-C, et al. 'Association between regional body fat and cardiovascular disease risk among postmenopausal women with normal body mass index'. *European Heart Journal* (2019) 40, 2849-2855 doi:10.1093/eurheartj/ehz391.

4 Pischon, T, M.D., et al. 'General and Abdominal Adiposity and Risk of Death in Europe'. *J Med*, N Engl 2008; 359:2105-2120 DOI: 10.1056/NEJMoa0801891.

5 Kekan, D, Kashalikar, S. 'Effect of Kapalbhati Pranayama on Waist and Hip Circumference'. *Journal of Evolution of Medical and Dental Sciences*, Researchgate 274881403. March 2013.

6 De Blasio A, et al. 'The Beneficial Effects of Essential Oils in Anti-Obesity Treatment'. *Int J Mol Sci.*, 2021 Oct 31;22(21):11832. doi: 10.3390/ijms222111832. PMID: 34769261; PMCID: PMC8584325.

7 Tokubuchi I, et al. 'Beneficial effects of metformin on energy metabolism and visceral fat volume through a possible mechanism of fatty acid oxidation in human subjects and rats'. *PLoS One.* 2017;12(2): e0171293. Published 2017 Feb 3. doi:10.1371/journal.pone.0171293.

8 Hurt RT, et al. 'L-arginine for the treatment of centrally obese subjects: a pilot study'. *J Diet Suppl.* 2014 Mar;11(1):40-52. doi: 10.3109/19390211. 2013.859216. Epub 2014 Jan 10. PMID: 24409974.

FIBROMYALGIA

1 Stefani Joanne Angelina Germanotta (born 1986), known as Lady Gaga, is an American singer, dancer, songwriter, and actress. She suffers from fibromyalgia, a condition affecting more than 6 million Americans. She has been dealing with what she calls "body pain, fear, paranoia, and anxiety for the past 5 years". Quote sourced from Van Meter, J. ' Lady Gaga Opens Up About A Star Is Born, MeToo, and a Decade in Pop'. *Vogue.com*, Sept 2018.

2 NHS. 'Fibromyalgia'. https://www.nhs.uk/conditions/fibromyalgia/.

3 Barber, S Dr., et al. House of Commons. 'Recognition of fibromyalgia as a disability'. Number CDP, 2019/0003. 14 January 2019.

4 McBeth, J. et al. 'Predictors of New-Onset Widespread Pain in Older Adults. Results From a Population-Based Prospective Cohort Study in the UK'. *Arthritis & Rheumatology*, Vol. 66, No. 3, March 2014, pp.757-767.

5 Moret C, Briley M. 'Antidepressants in the treatment of fibromyalgia'. *Neuropsychiatr Dis Treat.* 2006;2(4):537-548. doi:10.2147/nedt.2006.2.4.537.

6 Hennard J. 'A protocol and pilot study for managing fibromyalgia with yoga and meditation'. *Int J Yoga Therap.* 2011;(21):109-21. PMID: 22398352.

7 Saraswati, SS. *Asana Pranayama Mudra Bandha*, Yoga Publications Trust, Munger, Bihar, India, 1996. Reprinted 2008 at Thomson Press ltd, New Delhi, p.23.

8 Hohmann C, et al. 'The benefit of a mechanical needle stimulation pad in patients with chronic neck and lower back pain: two randomized controlled pilot studies'. *Evid Based Complement Alternat Med.* 2012; 2012:753583. doi: 10.1155/2012/753583. Epub 2012 Sep 11. PMID: 22997531; PMCID: PMC3446809.

9 Volker B, MD, et al. 'The Effect of Deep and Slow Breathing on Pain Perception, Autonomic Activity, and Mood Processing–An Experimental Study, *Pain Medicine*, Volume 13, Issue 2, February 2012, Pages 215-228.

10 Science Daily. Expert answer. 'Spike mat does help - a little, Swedish research shows'. Retrieved March 26, 2023.

11 Wiffen, P, et al. 'Carbamazepine for chronic neuropathic pain and fibromyalgia in adults'. *The Cochrane database of systematic reviews* (2014), 4. CD005451. 10.1002 /14651858.CD005451.pub3.

12 Goodin BR, et al. 'Oxytocin - a multifunctional analgesic for chronic deep tissue pain'. *Curr Pharm Des.* 2015;21(7):906-13. doi: 10.2174/1381 612820666141027111843. PMID: 25345612; PMCID: PMC4276444.

13 . Martin, M, et al. 'Cannabis-based medicines for chronic neuropathic pain in adults'. Authors' declarations of interest. Version published: 07 March 2018.

14 Nascimento SS, et al. 'Cyclodextrin-Complexed Ocimum basilicum Leaves Essential Oil Increases Fos Protein Expression in the Central Nervous System and Produce an Antihyperalgesic Effect in Animal Models for Fibromyalgia'. *International Journal of Molecular Sciences.* 2015; 16(1):547-563.

FLATULENCE

1 Martin Luther (1483–1546) was a German priest, theologian, author and professor, and Augustinian friar. He is the seminal figure of the Protestant Reformation whose followers became known as Lutherans. Quote sourced from AZquotes.com.

2 Saraswati, SS. *Asana Pranayama Mudra Bandha.* Yoga Publications Trust, Munger, Bihar, India, 1996. Reprinted 2008 at Thomson Press ltd, New Delhi, p.45.

3 Manzoor A, et al. 'Foeniculum vulgare: A comprehensive review of its traditional use, phytochemistry, pharmacology, and safety'. Indian Institute of Integrative Medicine (CSIR, IIIM), Sanat Nagar, Srinagar 190 005, India. Department of Chemistry, University of Kashmir, Hazratbal, Srinagar 190 006, India.

4 Markowiak P, Śliżewska K. 'Effects of Probiotics, Prebiotics, and Synbiotics on Human Health'. *Nutrients*, 2017 Sep 15;9(9):1021. doi: 10.3390/nu9091021. PMID: 28914794; PMCID: PMC5622781.

GETTING OLD

1 Ruth Elizabeth "Bette" Davis (1908– 1989) was an American actress with a career spanning more than 50 years. She was known for her forceful and intense style of acting. Quote sourced from Goodreads.com.

2 Underwood, B. 'Helen Mirren: "I Take Great Issue with the Term Anti-Aging"' www.oprahdaily.com

3 Kelder, P. *The Ancient Secret of the Fountain of Youth*, Virgin Books, 2011.

4 Sivaramakrishnan, D. et al. 'The effects of yoga compared to active and inactive controls on physical function and health related quality of life in older adults- systematic review and meta-analysis of randomised controlled trials'. *Int J Behav Nutr Phys Act* 16, 33 (2019).

5 Yamamoto K, et al. 'Poor trunk flexibility is associated with arterial stiffening'. *PubMed Am J Physiol Heart Circ Physiol*, 2009 Oct;297(4):H1314-8. doi: 10.1152/ajpheart.00061.2009. Epub 2009 Aug 7. PMID: 19666849.

6 MacDougall, D. 'The Soul: Hypothesis Concerning Soul Substance Together with Experimental Evidence of The Existence of Such Substance'. *American Medicine*, April 1907.

7 Khan S, Chang R. 'Anatomy of the vestibular system: A review'. *Neurorehabilitation*, (2013), 32 (3), 437-443.

8 The Five Tibetans. 'Which Direction Should I Spin?' t5t.com, June 2019.

9 Kelder, P. *Die Fünf Tibeter*, p.41, Der sechste Ritus, Scherz Verlag Bern 1999.

10 Epel E, et al. 'Can meditation slow rate of cellular aging? Cognitive stress, mindfulness, and telomeres'. *Ann N Y Acad Sci.*, 2009 Aug;1172:34-53. doi: 10.1111/j.1749-6632.2009.04414.x. PMID: 19735238; PMCID: PMC3057175.

11 Forbes MK, et al. 'Sexual Quality of Life and Aging: A Prospective Study of a Nationally Representative Sample'. *J Sex Res.* 2017 Feb;54(2):137-148. doi: 10.1080/00224499.2016.1233315. Epub 2016 Oct 31. PMID: 27798838; PMCID: PMC5235964.

12 Gad, MZ. 'Anti-aging effects of L-arginine', *Journal of Advanced Research*, Volume 1, Issue 3, 2010, pp.169-177, ISSN 2090-1232.

13 Jatoi S, et al. 'Low Vitamin B12 Levels: An Underestimated Cause Of Minimal Cognitive Impairment And Dementia'. *Cureus.* 2020 Feb 13;12(2):e6976. doi: 10.7759/cureus.6976. PMID: 32206454; PMCID: PMC7077099.

14 World Economic Forum. 'Want to live a long, healthy life? 6 secrets from Japan's oldest people', Sept. 2021.

HAIR LOSS

1 Gabrielle Bonheur "Coco" Chanel (1883-1971) was a pioneering French fashion designer. Her extraordinary influence on haute couture was such that she was the only person in the field to be named on *Time Magazine*'s 100 most influential people of the 20th century. Quote sourced from Goodreads.com.

2 Srivasyava, R. 'I understand why my patient is scared to lose her hair: it signals the loss of life, as she knows it'. *The Guardian*, June 2020.

3 Hunt N, McHale S. 'The psychological impact of alopecia'. *BMJ*, 2005 Oct 22;331(7522):951-3. doi: 10.1136/bmj.331.7522.951. PMID: 16239692; PMCID: PMC1261195.

4 Williamson D, et al. 'The effect of hair loss on quality of life'. *J Eur Acad Dermatol Venereol.* 2001 Mar;15(2): 137-9. doi: 10.1046/j.1468-3083.2001.00229.x. PMID: 11495520.

5 Choi S, et al. 'Corticosterone inhibits GAS6 to govern hair follicle stem-cell quiescence'. *Nature.* 2021 Apr;592 (7854):428-432. doi: 10.1038/s41586-021-03417-2. Epub 2021 Mar 31. PMID: 33790465; PMCID: PMC8923613.

6 Gupta, A. 'Can rubbing your nails together really improve your health? Here's your answer '. Healthshots, May 2021.

7 English RS Jr., Barazesh JM. 'Self-Assessments of Standardized Scalp Massages for Androgenic Alopecia: Survey Results'. *Dermatol Ther (Heidelb)* 2019 Mar;9(1):167-178. doi: 10.1007/s13555-019-0281-6. Epub 2019 Jan 22.

8 Dinh QQ, Sinclair R. 'Acupressure mat: Does it work? Female pattern hair loss: current treatment concepts. *Clin Interv Aging.* 2007;2(2):189-99. PMID: 18044135; PMCID: PMC2684510.

9 Fabbrocini G, et al. 'Female pattern hair loss: A clinical, pathophysiologic, and therapeutic review'. *Int J Womens Dermatol.* 2018 Jun 19;4(4): 203-211. doi: 10.1016/ j.ijwd.2018.05.001. PMID: 30627618; PMCID: PMC6322157.

10 Hay IC, MRCP, et al. 'Randomized Trial of Aromatherapy: Successful Treatment for Alopecia Areata | Complementary and Alternative Medicine'. *JAMA Dermatology,* JAMA Network. FRCPArch Dermatol. 1998;134(11):1349-1352. doi:10.1001/ archderm.134.11.1349.

11 Mooventhan A, Nivethitha L. 'Scientific evidence-based effects of hydrotherapy on various systems of the body'. *N Am J Med Sci.* 2014 May;6(5):199-209. doi: 10.4103/1947-2714.132935. PMID: 24926444; PMCID: PMC4049052.

12 Choi BY. 'Hair-Growth Potential of Ginseng and Its Major Metabolites: A Review on Its Molecular Mechanisms'. *Int J Mol Sci.* 2018;19(9):2703. Published 2018 Sep 11. doi:10.3390/ ijms19092703.

13 Ishida, W, et al. 'Severe Hair Loss of the Scalp due to a Hair Dye Containing Para phenylenediamine'. *ISRN Dermatol.,* 2011; 2011: 947284.

HANGOVERS

1 Winston Churchill (1874–1965), a famous British politician, was said sto have drunk 42,000 bottles of Champagne during his lifetime. He claimed it was one of life's essentials. Quote sourced from Goodreads.com.

2 Science Daily. 'Older drinkers may experience fewer hangovers than youngsters'. *Alcoholism: Clinical & Experimental Research Summary,* September 12, 2013.

3 Bhattacharya, A. 'Financial Headache. The cost of workplace hangovers and intoxication to the UK economy'. Institute of Alcohol Studies, 2019.

4 Roberts C, Robinson SP. 'Alcohol concentration and carbonation of drinks: the effect on blood alcohol levels'. *PubMed,* May 2016.

5 George, WH, et al. 'Indirect Effects of Acute Alcohol Intoxication on Sexual Risk-taking: The Roles of Subjective and Physiological Sexual Arousal'. *Arch Sex Behav* 38, 498–513 (2009).

6 Shakespeare, W. *Macbeth,* Act 2, Scene 3.

7 Varney E, Buckle J. 'Effect of Inhaled Essential Oils on Mental Exhaustion and Moderate Burnout: A Small Pilot Study'. *The Journal of Alternative and Complementary Medicine,*14 Jan 2013.

8 McMenamin, M. 'The Myth of Churchill and Alcohol: A Distortion of the Record'. The Churchill Project, May 18, 2018.

9 Quirynen M, et al. 'Impact of tongue cleansers on microbial load and taste'. *J Clin Periodontol.,* 2004 Jul;31(7):506-10.

10 Rangboo V, et al. 'The Effect of Artichoke Leaf Extract on Alanine Aminotransferase and Aspartate Aminotransferase in the Patients with Non-alcoholic Steatohepatitis Clinical Study' *Open Access* Volume 2016 |Article ID 4030476.

11 Coppersmith V, et al. 'The use of N-acetylcysteine in the prevention of hangover: a randomized trial'. *Sci Rep* 11, 13397 (2021). https://doi. org/10.1038/s41598-021-92676-0.

HAPPINESS

1 Ricky Dene Gervais (born 1961) is an English comedian, actor, director and writer. He co-created, co-wrote and acted in several British TV shows, including 'Afterlife', a love story , where he plays the main character, a widower who lost happiness after his wife has died. Quote sourced from Facebook, 9 July 2022.

2 Office for National Statistics. 'Estimates of life satisfaction, feeling that the things done in life are worthwhile, happiness and anxiety at the UK, country, regional, county and local authority level.' Oct 2021.

3 McRaven, WH. *Make Your Bed:*

Little Things That Can Change Your Life ...And Maybe the World. Grand Central Publishing, May 2017.

4 Merikanto I, et al. 'Evening types are prone to depression'. Chronobiol Int. 2013 Jun;30(5):719-25. doi: 10.3109/07420528.2013.784770. Epub 2013 May 20. PMID: 23688117.

5 Shevchuk, NA. 'Adapted cold shower as a potential treatment for depression'. Molecular Radiobiology Section, The Department of Radiation Oncology, Richmond, USA

6 American Associaties, Ben-Gurion University of the Negev. 'Hand-clapping songs improve motor and cognitive skills, research shows'. 3 May 2010.

7 Marmolejo-Ramos F, et al. 'Your face and moves seem happier when I smile. Facial action influences the perception of emotional faces and biological motion stimuli'. *Exp Psychol.,* 2020 Jan;67(1):14-22. doi: 10.1027/1618-3169/a000470.Epub 2020 May 11.

8 Strean WB. 'Laughter prescription'. *Can Fam Physician.* 2009;55(10):965-967.

9 Duberg A, et al. '"I feel free": Experiences of a dance intervention for adolescent girls with internalizing problems'. *Int J Qual Stud Health Well-being.* 2016;11:31946. Published 2016 Jul 12. doi:10.3402/qhw. v11.31946.

10 Dfarhud D, et al. 'Happiness & Health: The Biological Factors-Systematic Review Article'. *Iran J Public Health.* 2014 Nov;43(11):1468-77. PMID: 26060713; PMCID: PMC4449495.

11 Nehlig A. 'The neuroprotective effects of cocoa flavanol and its influence on cognitive performance'. Br *J Clin Pharmacol.* 2013;75(3):716-727. doi:10. 1111/ j.1365-2125.2012.04378.

12 Turakitwanakan W, et al. 'Effects of mindfulness meditation on serum cortisol of medical students'. J *Med Assoc Thai.* 2013 Jan; 96 Suppl 1:S90-5. PMID: 23724462.

13 Translation by Douglas Brooks from the *Upanishads*. A new translation by Vernon Katz and Thomas Egenes.

14 Hoenen M, et al. 'Fancy Citrus, Feel Good: Positive Judgment of Citrus Odor, but Not the Odor Itself, Is Associated with Elevated Mood during Experienced Helplessness'. *Front Psychol.,* 2016;7:74. Published 2016 Feb 2. doi:10.3389/ fpsyg.2016.00074.

15 Cheng Z, Smyth R. 'Sex and Happiness'. *Journal of Economic Behavior & Organization,* Vol. 112 April 2015, pp26-32, https://doi. org/10.1016/j.jebo.2014.12.030.

INSOMNIA

1 Charlotte Brontë (1816–1855), English novelist was the eldest of the three Brontë sisters, whose novels became classics of English literature. Even though she survived some of her siblings, her health was fragile, complaining of crushing insomnia, a poor appetite, grief and flashbacks. Quote sourced from Dominus, S. 'Overlooked No More: Charlotte Brontë, Novelist Known for 'Jane Eyre'. *The New York Times*.

2 von Schantz, M, et al. 'Associations between sleep disturbances, diabetes, and mortality in the UK Biobank cohort: A prospective population-based study'. *J Sleep Res.,* 2021; 30:e13392.

3 NICE. 'Insomnia: How common is it?' cks.nice.org, May 2022.

4 Lastella C, et al. 'Sex and Sleep: Perceptions of Sex as Sleep Promoting Behaviour in the General Adult Population'. *Frontiers in Public Health,* March 2019, 7. DOI: 10.3389/ fpubh.2019.00033.

5 Wang, WL, et al. 'The effect of yoga on sleep quality and insomnia in women with sleep problems: a systematic review and meta-analysis'. *BMC Psychiatry* 20, 195 (2020). https://doi.org/10.1186/s12888-020-02566-4.

6 Aulinas A, Arendt J. 'Physiology of the Pineal Gland and Melatonin'. Updated Oct 2022. https://www.ncbi.nlm.nih.gov/books/NBK550972/.

7 Datta K, et al. 'Yoga Nidra: An innovative approach for management of chronic insomnia - a case report'. *Sleep Science Practice* 1, 7 (2017). https://doi.org/10.1186/s41606-017-0009-4.

8 Gammoh O, et al. 'Chlorpheniramine, and escitalopram: Similar antidepressant and nitric oxide lowering roles in a mouse model of anxiety'. *Biomed Rep.* 2017; 6(6): 675-680. Doi: 10.3892/br.2017.901.

9 Gottesmann, C. 'GABA mechanisms and sleep'. *Review.* 2002;111(2):231-9. doi: 10.1016/s0306-4522(02)00034-9.

10 Koob GF, Colrain IM. 'Alcohol use disorder and sleep disturbances: a feed-forward allostatic framewor'. *Neuropsychopharmacology,* 2020 Jan;45(1):141-165. doi: 10.1038/s41386-019-0446-0. Epub 2019 Jun 24. PMID: 31234199; PMCID: PMC6879503.

11 Djokic G, et al. 'The Effects of Magnesium/Melatonin/Vit B Complex Supplementation in Treatment of Insomnia'. *Macedonian journal of medical sciences* vol. 7,18 3101-3105.30 Aug. 2019, doi: 10.3889/oamjms.2019.771.

12 Lee IS, Lee GJ. 'Effects of lavender aromatherapy on insomnia and depression in women college students'. Taehan Kanho Hakhoe Chi. 2006 Feb;36(1):136-43. Korean. doi: 10.4040/jkan.2006.36.1.136. PMID: 16520572.

MENOPAUSE

1 Julie Graham (born 1965) is a Scottish television and film actress. She has been developing a series that follows the life of women, who also happen to be going through the menopause. 'Dun Breedin' is available on YouTube and intends to change the representation of menopause. Quote sourced from Cherrington-Cook, J. 'Julie Graham talks menopause symptoms: 'I thought I was losing my mind'. YahooLife!, May 2020.

2 Wharton W, et al. 'Neurobiological Underpinnings of the Oestrogen - Mood Relationship'. *Curr Psychiatry Rev.,* 2012;8(3):247-256.doi:10.2174/157340012800792957.

3 Local Government Association. 'Menopause factfile'. local.gov.uk.

4 Cancer research. 'Does hormone replacement therapy (HRT) increase cancer risk?' https://www.cancerresearchuk.org/about-cancer/causes-of-cancer/hormones-and-cancer/does-hormone-replacement-therapy-increase-cancer-risk.

5 Jonasson AF, et al. 'Topical oxytocin reverses vaginal atrophy in post-menopausal women: a double-blind randomized pilot study'. *Menopause Int.,* 2011 Dec;17(4):120-5. doi: 10.1258/mi.2011.011030. Epub 2011 Nov 25. PMID: 22120944.

6 Rinpoche, T. 'The Practice of Sangha... Thich Nhat Hanh explains that sangha is more than a community, it's a deep spiritual practice'. Tsemrinpoche.com, April 2016.

7 Gould DC, Petty R. 'The male menopause: does it exist? Some men need investigation and testosterone treatment'. *West J Med.,* 2000;173(2):76-78. doi:10.1136/ewjm.173.2.76.

8 Afonso RF, et al. 'Yoga increased serum oestrogen levels in post-menopausal women – a case report'. *Menopause,* 2016 May; 23(5):584-6. doi: 10.1097/GME.0000000000000593. PMID: 26926324.

9 Nayak G, et al. 'Effect of yoga therapy on physical and psychological quality of life of perimenopausal women in selected coastal areas of Karnataka, India'. *J Midlife Health.,* 2014;5(4):180-185. doi:10.4103/0976-7800.145161.

10 Saraswati, SS. *Asana Pranayama Mudra Bandha*, Yoga Publications Trust, Munger, Bihar, India, 1996. Reprinted 2008 at Thomson Press ltd, New Delhi, p.60.

11 Eyre HA, et al. 'A randomized controlled trial of Kundalini yoga in mild cognitive impairment'. *Int Psychogeriatr.*, 2017;29(4):557-567. doi:10.1017/S1041610216002155.

12 Zope SA, Zope RA. 'Sudarshan kriya yoga: Breathing for health'. *International Journal of Yoga*, 2013, 6(1), 4-10. https://doi.org/10.4103 /0973-6131.105935.

13 Hooper L, et al. 'Effects of soy protein and isoflavones on circulating hormone concentrations in pre- and post-menopausal women: a systematic review and meta-analysis'. *Hum Reprod Update*, 2009 Jul-Aug;15(4):423-40. doi: 10.1093/ humupd/dmp010. Epub 2009 Mar 19. PMID: 19299447; PMCID: PMC2691652.

14 Williamson J, et al. 'Randomised controlled trial of reflexology for menopausal symptom's. *BJOG*, 2002 Sep;109(9):1050-5. doi: 10.1111/ j.1471-0528.2002.01504.x.PMID: 12269681.

15 Gröber U, et al. 'Magnesium in Prevention and Therapy'. *Nutrients.* 2015;7(9):8199-8226. Published 2015 Sep 23. doi:10.3390/nu7095388.

16 Poly C, et al. 'The relation of dietary choline to cognitive performance and white matter hyperintensity in the Framingham Offspring Cohort'. *Am J Clin Nutr.* 2011;94(6):1584-1591 doi:10.3945/ ajcn.110.008938.

17 Propper RE, et al. 'Correction: Getting a Grip on Memory: Unilateral Hand Clenching Alters Episodic Recall'. PLOS ONE, 2013, 8(5): 10.1371/annotation/693ff849-c230- 4e59-8772-b8755daf0f75.

OSTEOPOROSIS

1 Queen Camilla (born 1947) is the second wife of Charles III. Queen Camilla who was interviewed by Gloria Hunniford for the BBC to mark World Osteoporosis Day, reflected on her own experience of witnessing her mother suffer with osteoporosis. Quote sourced from Wylie, C. 'Camilla's stark warning to the young about osteoporosis'. *The Standard*, Oct 2021.

2 Svedbom A, et al. 'Osteoporosis in the European Union: a compendium of country-specific reports'. *Arch Osteoporosis.* 2013;8(1-2): 137. doi: 10.1007/s11657-013-0137-0. Epub 2013 Oct 11. PMID: 24113838; PMCID: PMC3880492.

3 Fishman, Loren M. MD, BPhil (Oxon) 'Yoga for Osteoporosis: A Pilot Study', *Topics in Geriatric Rehabilitation*: July-Sept 2009, Volume 25, Issue 3, pp244-250doi: 10.1097/TGR.0b013e3181b02dd6

4 Yang Y, et al. 'Long-term Proton Pump Inhibitor Therapy and Risk of Hip Fracture'. *JAMA*, 2006; 296(24): 2947-2953. doi:10.1001/ jama.296.24.2947.

5 Huovinen, V, et al. 'Bone mineral density is increased after a 16-week resistance training intervention in elderly women with decreased muscle strength'. *European Journal of Endocrinology* doi.org/10.1530/ EJE-16-0521, Vol. 175: Issue 6 Page Range: lit 571–582, Dec 2016.

6 van Ballegooijen AJ, et al. 'The Synergistic Interplay between Vitamins D and K for Bone and Cardiovascular Health: A Narrative Review'. *Int J Endocrinol.* 2017;2017:7454376. doi:10.1155/2017/7454376.

7 Civitelli R, Villareal DT, Agnusdei D, Nardi P, Avioli LV, Gennari C. Dietary L-lysine and calcium metabolism in humans. Nutrition. 1992 Nov- Dec;8(6): 400-5. PMID: 1486246

8 Harvard Health Publishing. 'Could too much calcium cause heart disease?' Harvard Medical School, August 2010, updated February 2020.

9 Tucker KL, et al. 'Colas, but not other carbonated beverages, are associated with low bone mineral density in older women: The Framingham Osteoporosis Study'. *Am J Clin Nutr.*, 2006 Oct; 84(4): 936-42. doi: 10.1093/ajcn/84.4.936. PMID: 17023723.

10 Katayama K, Matsuno T. 'Effects of bisphosphonates on fracture incidence and bone metabolism in rheumatoid arthritis patients in general practice taking long-term corticosteroid therapy: a retrospective study'. *Clin Drug Investig.* 2008; 28(3): 149-58. doi: 10.2165/00044011-200828030-00002. PMID: 18266400.

PANIC ATTACKS

1 Laurence, E. 'Ellie Goulding: How Fitness Helped Me Overcome Panic Attacks and Anxiety'. *Well+Good*, March 2017. British singer/songwriter Ellie Goulding (born 1986), has often spoken out about her battles with 'paralysing' anxiety attacks and about how she uses fitness to overcome panic attacks and anxiety.

2 Mind. 'What is a panic attack?' www.mind.org.uk.

3 Vassilev G, Hamilton, M. 'Personal and economic well-being in Great Britain'. Office for National Statistics, May 2021.

4 Slee, A, et al. 'Trends in generalised anxiety disorders and symptoms in primary care: UK population-based cohort study'. *The British Journal of Psychiatry* (2020) Page 1 of 7. doi: 10.1192/bjp.2020.159.

5 McLean CP, et al. 'Gender differences in anxiety disorders: prevalence, course of illness, comorbidity, and burden of illness'. *J Psychiatr Res.* 2011 Aug; 45(8):1027-35. doi: 10.1016/j.jpsychires. 2011.03. 006. Epub 2011 Mar 25. PMID: 21439576; PMCID: PMC3135672.

6 Ma X, et al. 'The Effect of Diaphragmatic Breathing on Attention, Negative Affect and Stress in Healthy Adults'. *Front Psychol.*, 2017 Jun 6;8:874. doi: 10.3389/fpsyg.2017.00874. PMID: 28626434; PMCID: PMC5455070.

7 NHS. 'Mindfulness'. https://www. nhs.uk/mental-health/self-help/tips-and-support/mindfulness/.

8 De Sousa DP, et al. 'A Systematic Review of the Anxiolytic-Like Effects of Essential Oils in Animal Models'. *Molecules* 2015, 20,18620-18660. doi. org/10.3390/molecules 201018620.

9 Todorov A,et al. (2017) 'Correlation between Depression and Anxiety and the Level of Vitamin B12 in Patients with Depression and Anxiety and Healthy Controls'. *Journal of Biomedical and Clinical Research*, Vol.10 (Issue 2), pp. 140-145. doi. org/10.1515/jbcr-2017-0023.

10 Boyle,NB, et al. 'The Effects of Magnesium Supplementation on Subjective Anxiety and Stress—A Systematic Review'.School of Psychology, University of Leeds, 26 April 2017, doi.org/10.3390/nu9050429.

11 Edge J. 'A pilot study addressing the effect of aromatherapy massage on mood, anxiety, and relaxation in adult mental health'. *Complement Ther Nurs Midwifery*, 2003 May;9(2):90-7. doi: 10.1016/S1353-6117(02)00104-X. PMID: 12697161.

12 Otte C. 'Cognitive behavioral therapy in anxiety disorders: current state of the evidence'. *Dialogues Clin Neurosci.* 2011;13(4):413-21. doi: 10.31887/DCNS.2011.13.4/cotte. PMID: 22275847; PMCID: PMC3263389.

13 Sancheza C, et al. 'A comparative review of escitalopram, paroxetine, and sertraline: are they alike?' *International clinical psychopharmacology* vol. 29,4 (2014): 185-96. doi:10.1097/YIC.0000000000000023.

QUEEFS

1 Tiffany Haddish (born 1979) is an American Emmy award-winning actress, comedian and author. She shared one of the things she wishes she would've learned about in her school health and sexual education class: queefing. Haddish says it was one of the most unexpected and embarrassing parts of sex for her, before she realised it was natural. Quote sourced from Lopez, C. ' Tiffany Haddish: Why teens should learn about queefing in sex ed'. *Business Insider India*, July 2020.

REFLUX

1 John Barrymore (1882–1942) was an American actor on stage, screen and radio. A heavy drinker, who eventually died because of liver cirrhosis, kidney failure and pneumonia. Quote sourced from picturequotes.com.

2 Revicki DA, et al. 'The impact of gastroesophageal reflux disease on health-related quality of life'. *Am J Med*. 1998 Mar;104(3):252-8. doi: 10.1016/s0002-9343(97)00354-9. PMID: 9552088.

3 Kamangar F, et al. 'Environmental causes of oesophageal cancer'. *Gastroenterol Clin North Am*. 2009;38(1):27-vii. doi:10.1016/j. gtc.2009.01.004.

4 Chen SH, et al. 'Is alcohol consumption associated with gastroesophageal reflux disease?' *J Zhejiang Univ Sci B*. 2010;11(6):423-428. doi:10.1631/jzus.B1000013.

5 'The Game Changers'. Watch this documentary and reconsider your eating habits. www.gamechangersmovie.com.

6 Hormone Health Network. 'Medicine Induced Bone Loss'. Hormone Health Network, Hormone. org, Endocrine Society, 21 June 2021.

SEX

1 Mary Jane West, "Mae West" (1893-1980). American actress, singer, playwright, screenwriter, and comedian, who was famous for her light-hearted wit and breezy sexual independence. Quote sourced from Quotefancy.com.

2 Loewenstein, G. et al. 'Does Increased Sexual Frequency Enhance Happiness?' *Journal of Economic Behavior & Organization*, 2015, 116.10.1016/j.jebo.2015.04.021.

3 YouGov. 'How often Brits have sex'. A weekly tracker of how many times in the past week, if any, you have had sex.

4 Brody S. 'The relative health benefits of different sexual activities'. *J Sex Med*. 2010 Apr;7(4 Pt 1):1336-61. doi: 10.1111/j.1743-6109.2009. 01677.x. Epub 2010 Jan 15. PMID: 20088868.

5 Study LH, et al. 'Is Sex Good for Your Health? A National Study on Partnered Sexuality and Cardiovascular Risk among Older Men and Women'. *J Health Soc Behav*. 2016;57(3):276-296. doi:10.1177/0022146516661597.

6 Joshi AM, et al. 'Role of Yoga in the Management of Premature Ejaculation'. *World J Mens Health*. 2020;38(4):495-505. doi:10.5534/ wjmh.190062.

7 Vikas D, et al. 'Yoga in Female Sexual Functions'. *The Journal of Sexual Medicine,* Vol. 7, Issue Part 2, February 2010, pp964-970.

8 Rosenblum, L. 'What is Tantra Yoga Really About?' Do You, March 2022, https://www.doyou.com/what-is-tantra-yoga-really-about/.

9 Meston, CM, et al. 'The Effects of Acute Exercise on Physiological Sexual Arousal in Women'. *Sex Hormones, Exercise and Women: Scientific and Clinical Aspects*. Cham: Springer International Publishing, 2023. 479-495.

10 Doty RL. 'Human Pheromones: Do They Exist?' *Neurobiology of Chemical Communication*. Boca Raton (FL): CRC Press/Taylor & Francis; 2014. Chapter 19.

11 Akhondzadeh S, et al. 'Efficacy and Safety of Oral Combination of Yohimbine and L-arginine (SX) for the Treatment of Erectile Dysfunction: a multicentre, randomized, double blind, placebo-controlled clinical trial'. *Iranian Journal of Psychiatry*, Winter 2010.

12 Lopresti AL, et al. 'A Randomized, Double-Blind, Placebo-Controlled,

Crossover Study Examining the Hormonal and Vitality Effects of Ashwagandha (Withania somnifera) in Aging, Overweight Males'. *Am J Men's Health*. 2019;13(2): 1557988319835985. doi:10. 1177/1557988319835985.

STRESS

1 Hans Selye (1907–1982) was a Canadian scientist, who conducted important scientific work on the hypothetical non-specific response of an organism to stressors. Quote sourced from Quotesgram.com.

2 Kirstin Aschbacher, et al. 'Good stress, bad stress and oxidative stress: Insights from anticipatory cortisol reactivity'. *Psychoneuroendocrinology*, Vol.38, Issue 9, 2013, pp1698-1708, ISSN 0306-4530, https://doi.org/10.1016/j. psyneuen.2013.02.004.

3 HSE. 'Work-related stress, anxiety, or depression statistics in Great Britain, 2022'. www.hse.gov.uk.

4 Statista. 'Most common types of stress experienced in the UK in 2020'. www.statista.com.

5 Crum AJ, Salovey P. 'Rethinking Stress: The Role of Mind-sets in Determining the Stress Response'. Department of Psychology, Yale University, February 25, 2013.

6 'Lynch J et al. 'Mantra meditation for mental health in the general population: A systematic review'. *European Journal of Integrative Medicine*. Volume 23, October 2018, pp101-108.

7 Jacobson E. 'The origins and development of progressive relaxation'. *Journal of Behaviour Therapy and Experimental Psychiatry*, Volume 8, Issue 2, June 1977, Pages 119-123.

8 Sharma VK, et al. 'Effect of fast and slow pranayama on perceived stress and cardiovascular parameters in young health-care students'. *Int J Yoga*, 2013 Jul;6(2):104-10. doi: 10.4103/0973-6131.113400. PMID: 23930028; PMCID: PMC3734635.

9 Chen MC, et al. 'The effects of aromatherapy in relieving symptoms related to job stress among nurses', *International Journal of Nursing Practice*, 2015, Wiley Online Library doi.org/10.1111/ijn.12229.

10 Cuciureanu MD, Vink R. 'Magnesium and stress'. Adelaide (AU): University of Adelaide Press; 2011.

TENNIS ELBOW

1 Copal, C. *A Bad Day at Tennis is Still Better Than a Good Day at Work*, Cassandra Copal notebooks, December 30, 2019.

2 Wetsman, N. 'Is it possible to be too flexible? Yoga might make you too bendy without making you strong enough to handle it'. *Popular Science*, Oct 2018.

3 Hohmann C, et al. 'The benefit of a mechanical needle stimulation pad in patients with chronic neck and lower back pain: two randomized controlled pilot studies'. *Evid Based Complement Alternat Med*. 2012;2012:753583. doi: 10.1155/2012/753583. Epub 2012 Sep 11. PMID: 22997531; PMCID: PMC3446809.

4 NHS. 'Tennis elbow'. www.nhs.uk/ conditions/tennis-elbow/treatment/.

5 Gosens, T, et al. 'Ongoing Positive Effect of Platelet-Rich Plasma Versus Corticosteroid Injection in Lateral Epicondylitis: A Double-Blind Randomized Controlled Trial With 2-year Follow-up'. *Am J Sports Med*., . 2011 Jun;39(6):1200-8.

6 Cogné M, et al. 'Number of botulinum toxin injections needed to stop requests for treatment for chronic lateral epicondylar tendinopathy. A 1-year follow-up study'. *Annals of Physical and Rehabilitation Medicine* Vol. 62, Issue 5, Sept. 2019, pp.336-341.

TINNITUS

1 Sir Richard Steele (1672 –1729), English essayist, dramatist and politician. Co-founder and principal author of *Tatler* and *The Spectator*. Quote sourced from Goodreads.com.

2 Ylikosi J, et al. 'Stress and Tinnitus; Transcutaneous Auricular Vagal Nerve Stimulation Attenuates Tinnitus-Triggered Stress Reaction'. *Front. Psychol.,* 17 September 2020, Vol 11, 2020 | https://doi.org/10.3389/fpsyg.2020.570196.

3 British Society of Audiology. 'The number of people living with tinnitus in the UK higher than previously thought'.March, 2019.

4 Köksoy S, et al. 'The Effects of Yoga in Patients Suffering from Subjective Tinnitus'. *Int Arch Otorhinolaryngol.,* 2018;22(1):9-13. doi:10.1055/s-0037-1601415 MLA.

5 Leaver AM, et al. 'Dysregulation of limbic and auditory networks in tinnitus'. *Neuron.* 2011 Jan 13;69(1):33-43. doi: 10.1016/j.neuron.2010.12.002. PMID: 21220097; PMCID: PMC3092532.

6 Singh C, et al. 'Therapeutic role of Vitamin B12 in patients of chronic tinnitus: A pilot study'. *Noise Health,* 2016;18(81):93-97. doi:10.4103/1463-1741.178485.

7 von Boetticher A. 'Ginkgo biloba extract in the treatment of tinnitus: a systematic review'. *Neuropsychiatr Dis Treat.,* 2011;7:441-447. doi:10.2147/NDT.S22793.

8 Jun HJ, Park MK. 'Cognitive behavioral therapy for tinnitus: evidence and efficacy'. *Korean J Audiol.,* 2013;17(3):101-104. doi:10.7874/kja.2013.17.3.101.

WEIGHT LOSS

1 Horwell, V. 'Jean Nidetch obituary'. *The Guardian,* 1 May 2015. The American business entrepreneur Jean Evelyn Nidetch (1923-2015) was the founder of Weight Watchers. Jean went from self-confessed 'fat housewife' to dieting evangelist with Weight Watchers International.

2 World Health Organization. 'WHO Regional Obesity Report 2022'.

3 Abdelaal M, et al. 'Morbidity and mortality associated with obesity'. *Ann Transl Med.,* 2017;5(7):161. doi:10.21037/atm.2017.03.107).

4 Sadokpam B, Bera, Dr TK. 'Effect of Yoga Exercises on Irisin Hormone in Obese People'. *International Journal of Health Sciences and Research.* https://www.ijhsr.org/IJHSR_Vol.8_Issue.6_June2018/25.pdf.

5 Epel E, et al. 'Stress may add bite to appetite in women: a laboratory study of stress-induced cortisol and eating behaviour'. *Psych neuroendocrinology,* 2001 Jan;26(1):37-49. doi: 10.1016/s0306-4530(00)00035-4. PMID: 11070333.

6 Pan WW, Myers MG Jr. 'Leptin and the maintenance of elevated body weight'. *Nat Rev Neurosci.* 2018 Feb;19(2):95-105. doi: 10.1038/nrn.2017.168. Epub 2018 Jan 11. PMID: 29321684.

7 Sutton et al. 'Early Time-Restricted Feeding Improves Insulin Sensitivity, Blood Pressure, and Oxidative Stress Even without Weight Loss in Men with Prediabetes'. *Cell Metabolism* 27, 1212-1221 June 5, 2018 ª 2018 Elsevier Inc.doi.org/10.1016/j.cmet.2018.04.010.

8 Lowe DA, et al. 'Effects of Time-Restricted Eating on Weight Loss and Other Metabolic Parameters in Women and Men with Overweight and Obesity: The TREAT Randomized Clinical Trial'. *JAMA Intern Med.,* 2020 Nov 1;180(11):1491-1499. doi: 10.1001/jamainternmed.2020.4153.

9 Dey S, Pahwa P. 'Prakriti and its associations with metabolism, chronic diseases, and genotypes: Possibilities of newborn screening and a lifetime of personalized prevention'. *J Ayurveda Integr Med.,* 2014;5(1):15-24.doi:10.4103/0975-9476.128848.

10 Jancy Rani, A, Dr. 'Effect of Bhastrika Pranayama on abdominal obesity in men and women - a randomized controlled trial'. The

Tamilnadu Dr.M.G.R. Medical University, Chennai, October 2019.

11 Elder RS, Mohr GS. 'The crunch effect: Food sound salience as a consumption monitoring cue'. *Food Quality and Preference*, Volume 51, 2016, pp.39-46, ISSN 0950-3293, https://doi.org/10.1016/j.foodqual.2016.02.015.

12 Hanh TN, Cheung L. *Savor: Mindful Eating, Mindful Life,* HarperOne, 2011.

13 Henley, J. 'Crisps: a very British habit'. *The Guardian*, Sept 2010.

14 Avena NM, et al. 'Evidence for sugar addiction: behavioural and neurochemical effects of intermittent, excessive sugar intake. *Neurosci Biobehav Rev.* 2008;32(1):20-39. doi:10.1016/j.neubiorev.2007.04.01.9

15 Elsawy G, et al. 'Effect of choline supplementation on rapid weight loss and biochemical variables among female taekwondo and judo athletes'. *J Hum Kinet.*, 2014 Apr 9;40:77-82. doi: 10.2478/hukin-2014- 0009. PMID: 25031675; PMCID: PMC4096089.

16 Diabetes Prevention Program Research Group. 'Long-term safety, tolerability, and weight loss associated with metformin in the Diabetes Prevention Program Outcomes Study'. *Diabetes Care,* 2012 Apr;35(4):731-7. doi: 10.2337/dc11-1299. PMID: 22442396; PMCID: PMC3308305.

APPENDIX

1 Ferretti, A. 'A beginner's guide to the chakras: channel more confidence, creativity, and joy in your life with a basic understanding of your body's energy centers'. *Yoga Journal,* 10 June 2021.

2 Phillips K, et al. 'Neuroscience and Neuropsychology Models of Brain based on Saint Amit Ray's 114-Chakra System'. *Neuropsyhcology Review J.* DO-10.13140/RG.2.2.26134.57927.

3 Tirtha SS. The *Ayurveda Encyclopedia. Natural Secrets to* Healing, *Prevention & Longevity,* Health Harmony. New Dehli. First edition 2006.

4 Fraser, T. *Live Better. Yoga exercises and inspirations for well-being.* Watkins Publishing Ltd. London. 2002.

FURTHER READING

The books listed here are the ones I found most inspiring and helpful throughout my yoga life and practice.

Coulter, David H., *Anatomy of Hatha Yoga*, Body and Breath, USA.

Fraser, Tara, *Yoga for You*, Watkins Publishing Ltd, London.

Frawley, David & Summerfield, Sandra, *Yoga for Your Type*, Lotus Press, USA.

Iyengar, B.K.S,. *Light on Yoga*, Thorsons, London.

Joy Devi, Nischala, *The Healing Path of Yoga*, Create Space Independent Publishing Platform.

Karmananda, Dr Swami, *Yogic Management of Common Diseases*, Yoga Publications Trust, India.

Kelder, Peter, *Die Fünf Tibeter*, translated by Christopher Baker, Scherz, Germany.

Folan Lilias M , *Lilias Yoga and You*, WCET-TV, Ohio, Cincinnati.

McCall, Timothy M.D. *Yoga as Medicine, A Yoga Journal Book* Bantam, USA.

Muktibodhananda, Swami, *Hatha Yoga Pradipika*, Bihar School of Yoga, India.

Saraswati, Swami Niranjanananda, *Prana Pranayama Prana Vidya*, Yoga Publications Trust, Bihar, India.

Swami Satyananda Saraswati, *Asana Pranayama Mudra Bandha*, Bihar School of Yoga, India.

Tirtha, Swami Sada Shiva, *The Ayurveda Encyclopedia*, Ayurveda Holistic Center Press.

INDEX

ABOUT THE AUTHOR

Carolin-Marie Roth, a former TV producer and presenter, has practised yoga for nearly 50 years and has been a British Wheel of Yoga teacher for more than 2 decades. Carolin's extensive experience means that she is lucky enough to have met, interviewed and taught many amazing and fascinating people. Her passion for living well through yoga is sincere and her classes are filled with laughter.

Carolin-Marie lives in Richmond-Upon-Thames, Surrey, with her husband, 3 daughters, 2 granddaughters and Bowie, the labradoodle.

Carolin-Marie Roth can be contacted at her Yoga Cube in Richmond, Surrey.
Email: Carolin@enjoyoga.co.uk
Instagram: @carolinmarie.yoga

ABOUT THE PHOTOGRAPHER

The artist and photographer Eva Lindner is my friend. A former ballet dancer, she shares my passion for perspective, movement and focus.

Eva meticulously stages her photos, crafting each frame with deliberate care. Beyond her technical prowess, Eva's photography resonates with a genuine warmth, authenticity, and a good sense of humour, which made me feel at ease in front of the camera.

Eva Lindner is based in Düsseldorf, Germany, where she lives with her husband, 5 children and 7 grandchildren. Instagram: @tanzeva5

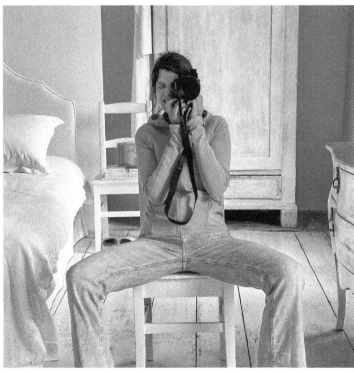

Photo by CM Roth

ACKNOWLEDGEMENTS

I am grateful to so many people for helping *Yoga, Sex and Happiness* come to life.

A huge thank you to my fellow yogi and editor Lesley Stonehouse, who read and corrected all the chapters more than once. I couldn't have done it without you Lesley!

To my friend Eva Lindner for taking the photos and being supportive and inspiring all the way.

Thank you to Emma, Tom and Dawn. You were an absolute pleasure to work with and I am so grateful to you for turning my dream into reality.

To Doris Zehr for inviting me into her beautiful home and photo location @anna-van-neerhave.de.

I would like to thank Fritzi, Riccarda and Paula for believing in me. Paula, thank you for your corrections and edits, you are a true star.

Jörg, thank you for your guidance, patience and encouragement. Love you.

Author Carolin-Marie Roth
Designers Emma Forge, Tom Forge
Editor Dawn Bates
Photographer Eva Lindner
Illustration Joey Gurdon
Jacket Design Emma Forge

First published in Great Britain in 2023 by
VDR Publishing, Richmond, London

10 9 8 7 6 5 4 3 2 1
001 Dec/2023

A CIP catalogue record for this book
is available from the British Library.
ISBN: 978-1-7384494-0-8

Warning
This book is not intended as a substitute for medical advice.
The publisher, author and the photographer cannot accept
any responsibility for any injuries or damage incurred because
of following the exercises in this book, or of using any of the
therapeutic methods described or mentioned. Before taking
any supplements, seek advice from your GP.

Printed in the USA
CPSIA information can be obtained
at www.ICGtesting.com
LVHW060323260124
769986LV00063B/908